To Love and Let Go

ALSO BY RACHEL BRATHEN

YOGA GIRL

to Love and Let Go

A MEMOIR OF LOVE, LOSS, AND GRATITUDE

RACHEL BRATHEN

G

GALLERY BOOKS

New York London Toronto Sydney New Delhi

G

Gallery Books
An Imprint of Simon & Schuster, Inc.
1230 Avenue of the Americas
New York, NY 10020

First Gallery Books trade paperback edition August 2021

GALLERY BOOKS and colophon are registered trademarks of
Simon & Schuster, Inc.

For information about special discounts for bulk purchases, please contact
Simon & Schuster Special Sales at 1-866-506-1949 or
business@simonandschuster.com.

The Simon & Schuster Speakers Bureau can bring authors to your live event.
For more information or to book an event, contact the Simon & Schuster
Speakers Bureau at 1-866-248-3049 or visit our website at
www.simonspeakers.com.

Interior design by Jaime Putorti

Manufactured in the United States of America

10 9 8 7 6 5 4 3 2 1

Library of Congress Cataloging-in-Publication Data has been applied for.

ISBN 978-1-5011-6399-9
ISBN 978-1-9821-1714-6 (pbk)
ISBN 978-1-5011-6400-2 (ebook)

To my mother, who is here
and my grandmother, who is not

And to Lea Luna,
who just arrived but was with us all along

CONTENTS

CONTENTS

To Love and
Let Go

1

THE END

It came out of nowhere. One minute I was standing with my boyfriend, Dennis, and our dog, Ringo, waiting for a flight, and the next I was on the floor, brought to my knees by a pain so fierce it felt as if someone had plunged a red-hot knife into my gut. I blacked out and woke up with my head in Dennis's lap. "What's happening?" he asked, his eyes filled with fear. I could barely speak. "My stomach," was all I could say. I tried to sit up but couldn't. The pain was making me dizzy. Someone called for help and, suddenly, paramedics appeared. My heart was okay, they said. Pulse: normal. Blood pressure: good. "Should we go to the hospital?" Dennis asked. I wanted to say yes. The stabbing pain I felt in my stomach was unlike anything I'd ever experienced in my life, and at twenty-five, I'd already been through quite a bit. *I should say yes*, I thought. *Something is definitely wrong. I should let him take me to the hospital.* "No," I said instead. "We can't miss our flight. Let's try to get to the gate."

It was a short flight, just thirty minutes from Aruba to Bonaire, where I was leading a yoga retreat that week. The retreat was sold out, with people coming from all over the world to see us. There was no way I was going to disappoint them. I was determined to get on the plane. Dennis helped me to my feet, but as soon as I stood up the invisible knife I felt plunged into my stomach twisted, and my knees buckled again. I knew what he was thinking. *This is crazy. We need a doctor.* He pleaded with me, but I wouldn't budge. "We have to get to Bonaire!" I said, looking at him sternly. "People are waiting for us."

It took all of my effort to get through passport control. I was too weak to hold on to anything but my boarding pass. I tried to put on a brave face, but on the inside I was terrified. *What is happening to me?* We made it to the gate and I collapsed into the nearest seat. My body was damp with sweat and my insides throbbed. Thinking I was going to vomit, I had to get to the bathroom. Hunched over, I made my way there but fell as I tried to open the stall door. Too weak to stand, I laid on the cold tile floor, curled up in a fetal position. *Am I dying?* Reaching into my purse for my phone to call Dennis for help, I heard a voice speak inside of me. "Get up. Keep moving. Get up." *Get up!* I told myself. *Get off the floor.*

I didn't even fully understand the urgency I felt about getting on the plane—was it really about not wanting to disappoint people, or was I trying to ignore whatever was happening to me? Whatever it was, I decided to keep going. I shoved my phone back into my bag, grabbed ahold of the wall, and pushed myself up to standing. When I looked in the mirror, a ghostly white face stared back, beckoning me to come to my senses and surrender. I was undeterred. *Move forward*, I told myself. *One step at a time.*

I made my way back to Dennis and Ringo and for the longest time we sat there, waiting to board. My stomach hurt so much it felt as if my insides were on fire. The hands on the clock crawled. Finally it was time. Approaching the flight attendant with my boarding pass, I watched her face twist in horror. "You can't fly!" she said. "You are obviously not well." I was pale, and my forehead was slick with sweat. I had a hard time focusing my gaze, but did my best to compose myself. "I'm going to Bonaire," I said. The flight attendant looked at me. "This plane is going to Bonaire," she said. "You, my dear, are not." I gritted my teeth in pain and frustration. I just wanted to get on the damn plane and settle in. "*I have to* get on," I said, pleading. "Please, I beg you. I'm okay—I promise. It's just a stomach bug. I'll be fine. I just have to get on this flight." I don't know why she finally gave in. "Will you seek medical attention when you get there?" she asked. Yes, I promised. "Go on, then," she said, pointing the way. "Hurry, before my manager sees you."

I expected to see a plane at the gate, but a shuttle bus idled there. The heat was sweltering and the bus was full. I couldn't bear the thought of even the short ride to our plane. Dennis climbed in first with Ringo and our baggage before lifting me up into the bus. I grabbed a handle and held tight. My long hair clung to my back, and I could feel sweat dripping off my face. Why was it so hot in here? As the engine roared, the urge to throw up overtook me. *I don't throw up.* It's at the very top of my list of things I can't handle. I hadn't done it since I was a teenager and chugged an entire bottle of vodka by myself. But there, on that bus, I felt it coming. I looked around frantically for a plastic bag, a bin, something. Anything. Could I will myself not to vomit until I was off the damn bus?

The moment the brakes squealed and the bus came to a stop, and before the doors were fully open, I pressed myself out of the shuttle. At the top of the stairs leading into the plane was the woman who'd taken my boarding pass. How did she make it there so quickly? She gave me a stern look. *If I throw up now*, I thought, *she isn't going to let me board*. In desperation, I walked behind the bus, bent over, and hurled my insides out all over the tarmac. Wiping my arm on my sleeve, I took the steps up to the plane and fell into my seat. The next thing I knew, I was waking up in a cab with Dennis and Ringo, racing to the emergency room in Bonaire. Bonaire is a tiny Caribbean island with fewer than nineteen thousand people. The hospital is so small that the maternity ward is connected to the hospice. You die where you're born. Two doctors treated me, both tall and Dutch looking. Poking and prodding my abdomen, they gave their diagnosis: a probable ruptured appendix. To be certain, they said, an ultrasound would have to be performed, but there was only one ultrasound specialist on the whole island and it would take time for him to get to me. Until then, I would be given morphine to make me more comfortable, the doctors said before disappearing.

The pain was unbearable. I had never experienced anything like it in my entire life. Where was the morphine? It had been hours. Did no one understand I was dying from the pain? I had reached a level of agony that I didn't think was possible.

Finally, a nurse appeared with a needle. They hooked me up to an IV and I sighed with anticipation as I watched the first dose of morphine drip into my arm. "Just breathe, honey," the nurse said. "The pain will be over in a minute."

I'd never experienced morphine, but from what I'd heard, and seen in movies, I expected fast relief. I writhed in pain, waiting for the reprieve, but it didn't come. Fifteen minutes later I was on my side, legs curled up, screaming. The doctors increased the dose. Still nothing. I was almost at a point of no return when the ultrasound technician arrived. By then, seven hours had passed since I first collapsed at the airport. "I hear you have a ruptured appendix," he said. "I need to do the ultrasound right away to make sure they don't put you through surgery for no reason."

Dennis held my hand as the technician applied a cold gel to my abdomen. I felt a strange sense of déjà vu. I had envisioned this before, I realized: Dennis holding my hand, both of us looking into a tiny monitor, ultrasound technician applying gel to my stomach . . . It felt familiar. Surely, I'd dreamt it. I'd known since the moment we met that one day Dennis and I would be parents. I wished I could catapult us into the future, to a moment other than this one; one where we were happy, waiting to hear the heartbeat of our future child. I'd do anything to not be here, panicked, trying to find out if whatever pain I was experiencing was going to kill me. Dennis squeezed my hand tightly. The technician pressed the device into my belly and started scanning. After a few minutes, he looked puzzled. "What's wrong?" Dennis asked. He'd never seen me like this. I'm a resilient person; I can manage pain. I could tell by the look on his face that he was terrified. "What is it? Is it worse than they thought?" The technician shook his head. "No," he said. "I can't . . . I can't find anything. There is no indication that anything is ruptured or even swollen. By the look of the scan, you are totally fine." I was stunned. "But, the pain," I said. "I know there is something seriously wrong. I feel like I'm going to die!"

The doctors couldn't understand it either—where was the pain coming from? Why didn't anything show on the ultrasound? And why wasn't the morphine working? Soon I was delirious. I saw visions. The pain came in waves like red-hot lava. It was all-consuming. The tallest of the two doctors came back, visibly worried. He no longer spoke directly to me but addressed Dennis. "We normally don't open people up without knowing what we are looking for, but the amount of pain she is in leaves us no choice," he said. "She will go into surgery in the morning. But she cannot stay in this state until then; she is dehydrated and the morphine isn't taking. I'd like to administer a huge dose of morphine, large enough to put her to sleep."

I heard him speaking, but I wasn't listening. The fire inside of me had taken over. I imagined the inside of my skin was sizzling, a dark mist oozing out of my abdomen. It was similar to my experience years earlier during an ayahuasca ceremony when I'd hallucinated frightening things. I remembered that I'd escaped that nightmare by letting go, by giving in to the fear of my own death. I didn't know if I was dying now, but it sure felt like it. I just knew I couldn't take the pain anymore. I felt Dennis gently shaking my shoulders to help me regain consciousness. "Babes," he said. "They are going to give you something to make you fall asleep. Okay? Morphine, a lot of it. To make the pain go away. But you won't be awake. Is that okay?" "Yes," I said, slurring. "Whatever they want. I'm going into the fire."

Minutes later the doctor came back and injected the medicine into my thigh. "Let go," he said. "Fall asleep." I closed my eyes. The flames started changing color from deep red and orange to pale yellow, then blue. Suddenly, my body took a deep, full breath. I could feel the inhale making space within me, clearing the fire that had been consuming my insides. As I exhaled, the pain disappeared. It was gone. Just like that. The feeling was indescribable. I was floating in a cool, quiet ocean. Everything was still and calm.

I'd begun to drift away when I heard a phone ringing in the background. *Who is calling?* I clung to consciousness, listening as Dennis rustled through my purse to find my phone. It was Luigi, one of my closest friends from Costa Rica. *He must have heard I was in the hospital*, I thought. *I'll just let him know I'm okay.* Dennis put the phone to my ear. "I'm okay," I said. "I'm in the hospital, but I'm okay. The pain is gone now." "Hospital?" Luigi said on the other end, sounding confused. There was something else in his voice, too, something I couldn't pinpoint. "Why are you in the hospital?" "I don't know," I said. I could hear myself slurring. "But it's okay now. Everything is okay." Luigi was quiet for a long time. When he spoke I could tell something wasn't right. I tried to stay awake so I could hear him. "Amor. I don't know how to tell you this. Fue un accidente. Con Andrea. Andrea tuvo un accidente." I couldn't comprehend Luigi's words. Why was he talking about Andrea? Andrea was my best friend. We hadn't spoken for a few days,

she was at a concert with her boyfriend. What was he saying?
Andrea had an accident?

A feeling of terror overcame me, but I wasn't able to grasp
it. It didn't feel real, but like something that was far, far away.
Andrea and I were soul mates. Sometimes it felt as if we were
the same soul living in two bodies. I didn't know where I
began and she ended. We felt each other's pain; read each
other's thoughts. I forced myself to speak. "What happened?
Can I talk to her?" I asked. "No," Luigi said. I heard him
swallow hard on the other end of the line. "Luigi. What is it?
Tell me," I urged him. My knuckles were white from clutching the phone so hard. He took a deep breath and finally
spoke. "Falleció." My heart froze. The room started spinning.
I dropped the phone onto the bed. "Can you talk to Luigi?"
I asked Dennis. "I'm too tired now." I turned on my side and
squeezed my eyes shut. I heard the echo of the word he'd
just said in my mind. *Falleció*. I am fluent in Spanish, but
that was a word I'd never used before. In my mind I knew
what it meant because I'd heard it, but right now, lying in a
hospital bed on a foreign island, I couldn't comprehend its
meaning. In my mind's eye I saw it spelled out in front of me.
F-A-L-L-E-C-I-Ó. Something terrifying was hiding behind
that word. I wasn't sure what it was. I decided I wasn't ready
for it. I'd think about it some other time. The ocean was pulling me away. I let it take me.

At some point during the night I woke up. Dennis was
sitting next to me, his head in his hands, crying. Dennis never
cries. There was that feeling again. Terror. Like a cloud, but far
away. Luigi's voice echoed in my head. *Falleció*. Fear gripped

my heart. *I don't want to be here*, I thought, closing my eyes. The ocean rolled in again. Beckoning me. I jumped in.

Suddenly, I am in a new place. It is a hospital but not in Bonaire. I'm standing in a hallway. Everything is blinding white. I'm wearing a hospital gown and pink lace underwear. A girl is standing at the far end of the corridor, twirling her dark hair between her fingertips. She turns toward me and I smile. Andrea! I walk toward her. She hugs me, and for the longest time we're just standing there, holding each other.

"I think something happened," I say. "I think I'm in the hospital."

"We are," Andrea says.

Something is wrong. I feel scared. When Andrea smiles, I feel calm again.

"Can you come stay with me?" I ask her. "I don't want to wake up alone."

"No," she says. "I can't stay. I have to go."

It seems ludicrous, that we are here in this hospital together but apparently in different rooms. We should push our beds together and I can read to her like we used to do when we were living in Dominical.

"Please don't leave," I say. Andrea's face is glowing. She looks so beautiful. I want to touch her.

"I'm here. I'm always right here," she says, but she is backing away.

I try to grab her hand but I can't reach it. The hallway is long and she is so far away that I can barely see her anymore. The light is blinding. I have to close my eyes. When I open them, she is gone.

Sunlight was streaming through the window in my room. There was a plastic bracelet with my name on it around my wrist. *Right*, I thought. *I'm in the hospital. In Bonaire.* I looked around the room and saw Dennis. His eyes were red. He took my hand. It looked like he was about to say something but he stopped himself. Then: "Do you remember much from last night?" he asked.

"What do you mean? The doctors?"

"No . . . Never mind," he said.

I wanted to ask him what he was about to say, but something stopped me.

"They are coming to get you for surgery soon," he said.

"Okay."

"We have to take your clothes off. And all your bracelets."

I had so many bracelets. Some I'd picked up on my travels, others were gifts. One was a friendship bracelet I shared with Andrea. Most were tied to my arm.

"The doctors say we have to cut these off," Dennis said.

He leaned in with a pair of scissors. "*No!*" I screamed. "I need these bracelets! You can't cut them off! Tell them I won't do the surgery if I have to cut them off."

"Okay," he said.

Dennis left the room and came back with a roll of gauze. "We can wrap up your wrist in this," he said. "You don't have to cut them."

"Good."

Time passed. I had drifted off again, only to be awakened by the attendants taking me to surgery.

Dennis leaned over and kissed me. "I'll be right here when

you get back, okay?" I was scared. Why was I having surgery? I couldn't remember. "I don't want it anymore," I said. "Please don't let them take me."

Tears filled Dennis's eyes. "Everything is okay," he said. "You're just going to be asleep for a little while and then you'll wake up and I'll be here."

"I think something has happened," I said.

Dennis looked at me. "We don't have to talk about it now. I love you."

I squeezed my eyes shut. When I opened them again I was in a sterile room, a bright white light shining overhead. Doctors hovered over me. Someone was taking off my hospital gown but stopped suddenly. "They didn't tell you that you had to take your underwear off?"

I looked down. I was naked, except for pink lace underwear.

It felt strange, almost dirty, my lace underwear in such a sterile room.

"We're going to have to cut them off."

"Okay."

The attendant covered my face with a mask. "Ten, nine, eight . . ." The ocean took me again.

When I woke up, the light was different. Dennis was by my side, just as he had promised. I put a hand on my stomach. Three balls of gauze were taped to my belly, covered in some sort of plastic. It felt raw and sore. Dennis held my hand. I looked at him. His eyes filled with tears. *Falleció.* The word was painted in thick black letters across my mind, letters dripping with a knowing I was not ready to face. *If I don't ask the question, I won't have to know the answer*, I thought. Instead, I asked Dennis what happened to me.

"Your appendix was inflamed. They removed it," he said.

"Oh."

He opened his mouth, about to continue, but stopped himself. There was so much pain in his eyes. The silence in the room was deafening. We were quiet for a long time.

"Where is Andrea?" I finally asked.

Tears ran down his cheeks. "There was a car accident," he said.

"Is she okay?"

I already knew the answer.

Dennis shook his head.

Falleció. The word stems from the intransitive verb *fallecer.* *Fallecer.* To pass away. To die.

Everything went black.

They told me later that I screamed. After the doctors had discussed the surgery with me, Dennis left the room to go to the bathroom. I reached for my phone and dialed Andrea's number. It went straight to voice mail. *Strange*, I thought. *I'll try her later.* It was only three months until my wedding and she still hadn't seen her bridesmaid's dress. It was hanging at my dad's place in Sweden, waiting for us all to arrive. Dusty blue. I'd made a chat group with my bridesmaids: Olivia, Rose, Jessica, Mathias (brides-man!), and Andrea. We were talking in the chat group every day, planning wedding details. It had taken us forever to decide between seafoam and dusty blue. Andrea wanted dusty blue. I dialed her number again. She didn't pick up.

I call Luigi. "Where is Andrea?" I ask. He is crying. "She was driving home from the beach," he says. She ended up on the wrong side of the road. A truck hit her head-on. It had taken her all day to die. They sent her to the wrong hospital twice. Everything went wrong. As he is speaking, I feel myself floating away. Is this what an out-of-body experience feels like? I am listening to his words but I'm not understanding him. None of this is real. None of this is actually happening. I try to listen to what he is saying but it's hard because what's the point in listening to words said in a dream you're about to wake up from any moment? Luigi keeps talking. I can tell it's important to him that he is the one sharing this with me; I can tell that he is choosing his words carefully. He says something about surgery and the hospital and the eight hours she fought for her life. Something about that last sentence jolts me back to reality. Eight hours? I do the math in my head and the realization that follows is so gut-wrenching it knocks the breath out of my lungs. During all of the hours I had just spent in agony, Andrea was dying. The moment I collapsed at the airport was the exact moment she hit the truck. That red-hot knife I felt stabbed into my gut was her pain, too. They operated on her stomach to stop the internal bleeding. Our pain came from the same place. Her heart stopped twice. They tried to revive her. It wasn't my pain. It was ours. It was hers.

The moment my pain went away, the moment I took that deep, full breath . . . was the moment Andrea took her last.

2
___

AWAKEN

I've known death since I was a little girl—my mother introduced us. On the day of my fifth-birthday party, she tried to
kill herself. It happened after a celebration with family and
balloons and cake and presents, and when the party was over,
she said she was tired and asked my dad to take my brother
and me home with him for the night. We were halfway to my
dad's house when he realized he'd left something behind (or
maybe he had a premonition), and we turned back. Mom was
near death when we got there. She'd swallowed two bottles
of sleeping pills chased by vodka. I didn't find the suicide letters until much later: one for family and friends, one for my
brother, one for me. *I love you so much and I am so sorry* . . . I
found the letters years later, tucked away neatly in a box in
the bottom of a drawer in our living room. There were pictures of me as a baby, old postcards, some drawings, and right
there among all the regular memories was an envelope marked
"Rachel." My hands shook as I opened it. I was twelve by

then, and as I sat on the floor reading my mother's final good-bye to me I remember thinking: *this is probably going to happen again.*

My parents met when they were very young. Mom was nineteen and waiting tables to make ends meet. Dad was four years older and already running several casinos and nightclubs in town. I remember asking my mom if she was ever truly in love with my dad. "I don't know," she said. "He gave me safety. And security. He wore these funny-looking suits. We never fought, but he worked all the time. I was always alone."

I was Mom's miracle baby, she said, because she was going through a dark time and having me saved her life. I heard that sentence more times than I could ever count as a child: *You saved my life.* My miracle, she'd say. *Mitt mirakel.* She soon discovered she was pregnant again, and I was two when my brother, Ludvig, was born. Not long after, my parents split up. Sweden is not a big country, but when Mom decided to study away from our home in Uppsala to become an air traffic controller, it meant I had to stay behind with dad for big parts of the week. She told me that, at one point, while she was away, my father tried to send my brother and me off to a boarding school in the States. Because, according to my mom, if *he* couldn't keep the family together, he didn't want her to have us either. Luckily, the nanny called her in a panic and she rushed home before he could get us to the airport. I don't know if it's true—looking back at my life, I realize there is so much that I don't know. My mother's version of events was always the complete opposite of my father's.

Mom was almost a year into her studies when she fell in love with another man, a fighter pilot named Stefan whom she'd met on the military base she was training at. We all moved in together, leaving my father behind. My brother and I started a new school, and my grandmother came to live with us for long stretches of time. I think my dad went insane with jealousy. My mother leaving him, then finding someone else, taking his kids to live with another man . . . It was all too much. He once described the move to me as a "kidnapping." He said he came to pick us up one day and we were just gone, and he had no idea where we went. That he looked for us everywhere; he wanted his kids back. I know when he finally found us he made our lives miserable. At one point he threatened Stefan's life, and Stefan started sleeping with his military weapon in his bedside table (in Sweden this is unheard-of—guns are not a part of our society). Dad's threats got so bad my mom started recording their phone calls in case she had to take him to court. The end result was that my mom got sole custody of us and, for a while, we lost touch with my dad.

Mom, Stefan, and I were on the couch watching a movie when I had my first-ever asthma attack. Stefan was the one who brought me to the hospital and held the oxygen mask over my face while I fought to breathe. It was only once I was an adult that I learned that asthma, though a physical and sometimes chronic illness, is emotionally connected to suppressed anger and fear. It wasn't strange that, while on the surface things looked good, I started to develop physical ailments. My parents had separated and very traumatically so. My family was broken. And I didn't know where my dad was anymore. What I remember most is that Mom was happy, so those other things

didn't actually matter all that much. It was the first time in
my life I'd seen her that way: genuinely happy. Peaceful. She
was happy, so I figured I should be happy, too. To me, Stefan
was like a real, live superhero. He flew planes, climbed mountains, and skied faster than anyone I knew. And he was always
smiling. That's what I remember most about him: his smile.
And the way he made my mom smile, too. One of my most
cherished childhood memories is sitting on Stefan's shoulders
at an après-ski during a ski trip in the north of Sweden. We'd
been on the slopes all day and Stefan used his ski to carve us a
little nest in the snow, where we sat on blankets, drinking hot
chocolate in the sun. I remember my mom happy, turning her
face toward the sun, wrapped in his arms.

Later at the hotel there was a band playing and we danced,
with me on his shoulders; Stefan holding my hands, making
sure I wouldn't fall. I was only four years old but I remember
that moment so clearly, feeling like I was on top of the world. I
have little snapshots of memories like that; they are all beautiful, warm, happy, but I can't piece them together. I do remember him smiling, all the time. It was only a few months after
that day on the slopes that our lives would change forever.

Mom and Stefan were about to be married and had just
bought a house together. A few days before they were to sign
the papers for the house she was giving my brother a bath when
our doorbell rang. I answered it to find Stefan's best friend and
flight partner, along with the captain of the air force, a psy-
chologist, and a priest standing there. While I went to play
in another room, the men informed Mom that, earlier that
morning, Stefan had flown his "Drake" (the Swedish word for

dragon), a high-speed military airplane, into the ocean during a training session. He was found dead outside the plane.

I don't remember opening the door. I don't remember being told to go play in another room. I don't know what happened to my brother—he was in the bath. Who held him? Who held me? Mom collapsed when she heard. I've had this story told to me so many times, but only remember bits and pieces of it myself. That's how trauma works—our minds shut down to protect us. Too much, too soon. I remember my grandmother taking me and my brother outside during the funeral, rushing us through the church aisle, covering our ears so we wouldn't have to hear our mother's wailing. I remember the little cards we were given, written in my mom's handwriting but signed by Stefan. These were the worst hours of her life, but she still managed to get creative to console us and wrote my brother and me letters in his name, explaining how much he loved us and that he would always live in our hearts. I remember a lot of family around, everyone with dark, sad faces. I was filled with questions and deep sadness, but I couldn't rely on Mom for answers; she was inconsolable. Barely there. I didn't want to add to her pain by telling her how upset I was. In the midst of all this trauma, no one ever sat me down to explain where Stefan had gone. Someone had mentioned that "he went to heaven"—but I knew that; he flew his plane in the sky all the time. I was almost five years old, which I think was old enough to make sense of some of it, but not old enough to fully understand. I asked a relative what happened to Stefan. She said, "Oh, honey, he loved you *so* much. He wanted to hurry home to see you, but he flew his plane too fast and it crashed in the ocean." She had only good intentions, but I understood that to mean it was my fault that Stefan had died. If he had only loved me a little less, I thought, he wouldn't have hurried back to see me, and he would still be alive and my mother would be okay. Instead, everything was dark and terrible. I'd lost my stepdad and my mom was so consumed with grief I could barely reach her anymore.

After that, we moved back to our hometown of Uppsala and I got to see my dad again. I ran to him and he picked me up. Slumping into his arms, I felt safe and allowed myself to cry, something I hadn't been able to do with my mom because it would have upset her. "Did you know Stefan died?" I asked. "Yes, I know," my father said. "And it is *good* that he died." Hearing his words, I froze. To this day my dad claims he never spoke those words, but I remember them clearly. He spoke from pain, from jealousy, from having spent more than a year blaming another man for taking his children away. At that moment I understood: there was no one I could talk to, no one I could trust. I had loved Stefan, but no one would give me permission to grieve. Not my dad, and certainly not my mom, whose own grief had caused her to become increasingly unstable as the days passed.

With time, visits from family members became more and more infrequent and, eventually, it was just the three of us again. Caring for my mother fell to me. In the mornings before school I got my little brother up before taking Mom her favorite breakfast in bed—coffee with milk, and bread with cheese and orange jam on a tray. I was just learning to read, but I already knew how to work the coffee machine. Mom was a ghost of her former self, barely functioning, which left me to pick up her motherly duties, things like holding Ludvig's hand when we crossed the street and blowing out the candles she lit in the evenings and left burning after she went to bed.

Her broken heart incapacitated my mother. For the longest time, when I couldn't sleep, I would lie facedown on the bed, put the pillow over the back of my head, and scream into the mattress, because that was what my mom did. I thought she did it to help her sleep. I didn't understand that her screams were those of unspeakable grief. I don't think the rest of the family knew how bad things were until she tried to take her own life on the day of my birthday party. She survived, but barely, and was committed to a psychiatric institution for a few weeks.

When she finally made it home, Mom tried to pick up the pieces and did her best to start her life again. She had lost her soul mate, her best friend, and her home in the blink of an eye; she had to start a whole new life all alone. I did my best to cheer her up, and after a while I decided that I would make it my sole purpose to get her to become happy again. I truly believed that if I just tried hard enough, I could make her better. That meant doing well in school, keeping myself clean and organized, and not making a fuss about anything. I did my best to be a good girl.

With time, she got healthy enough to take a job in Stockholm at a consulting firm, an hour from our house in Uppsala. She was a single mom, commuting for hours every day and working hard to get by. My brother and I were always the last kids to get picked up from "fritids," the after-school activity center. The teachers often stayed late with us, waiting for my mother to arrive. I loved being the last one there, helping the teachers turn all the lights off and putting everything away.

My dad, meanwhile, established a life for himself an hour's flight away in Riga, Latvia, on the shores of the Baltic Sea. We rarely saw him after he moved away. I was eight when, out of the blue, he called to say he was having a daughter with a Ukrainian woman named Natasha, but before the baby was born, he left Natasha for an even younger woman named Inga. Dad didn't see the baby much, but when I visited him I always went to see her. Her name was Katja and she was beautiful. I loved the idea of having a half sister. It made me feel less alone.

While Dad was busy trying to keep up with his much younger girlfriend, my mom met Calle, a handsome, bearded sailor from Stockholm. They fell in love, or so I think. I don't know what kind of love is possible when you've just lost your soul mate. I can only imagine. I do know I liked Calle, and didn't mind having him around. After a little while Mom got pregnant and we moved in with Calle and his daughter from a previous marriage, who lived with us every other week. Living in Stockholm was different. I was so nervous to start school I could barely sleep the whole week before. What if nobody liked me? What if I didn't fit in? The day before school was to begin I fell on a railing and broke a bone in my hand. I had to go to school with a cast on and the mere thought of it made me mortified. I didn't want to attract any attention, and now I'd have to show up with my arm in a sling! Turns out, the broken bone was a godsend. I made friends on the first day—everyone wanted to know how I'd gotten the cast and what had happened.

Mom gave birth to my little sister Hedda when Katja was a year old. Now I had two half sisters. I loved Hedda an unbelievable amount—she was so little and so fragile, and she needed me. I took it upon myself to care for her as much as I could. I learned how to change her diapers, and how to dance around the kitchen with her when she was fussy and didn't want to sleep. Even though I was only ten, sometimes it felt like Hedda was mine.

Life was pretty stable for a while. Our new family had settled in and Dad even visited occasionally to take me to dinner, or shopping for a new winter jacket, or to go on ski weekends. Mom and Calle seemed happy enough, but apparently all was not well because, when Hedda was just seven months old, Mom left him for her coworker, who was named, serendipitously, Stefan. Life was about to turn upside down again.

Mom moved us from Calle's place into a new apartment with Stefan in a nice part of Stockholm. It was huge, with five bedrooms, big enough for the three of us kids and his twins from a previous marriage. They soon married, but I don't remember much of the ceremony, except that when they said their vows, rather than repeating after the priest and saying, "I promise to love and cherish you for as long as I live," my mother said, "I want to love and cherish you for as long as I live." Looking back at it now, I know she really did want to promise, she just couldn't. She lost something when Stefan died and I don't think she knew how to get it back. That same year, my dad married Inga in a much more extravagant ceremony. I gave a speech in front of 275 people. "The year 2000 was the year my parents finally got married," I said. "But not to each other." The crowd laughed.

Within months, both sets of parents were expecting. My two new baby sisters were born within three months of each other: Emelie to Dad and Inga in May of 2001 and Maia to Mom and Stefan that same August. The whirlwind of events meant an abrupt change in my family tree. Now I had an ex-stepsister I didn't see anymore, two new stepsiblings, four half sisters, and, of course, my brother. If that wasn't enough to send me reeling, Mom and Stefan had decided to move us out of the city to a big white house on the nearby island of Lidingö.

I didn't want to go. I was growing into my own and had only recently realized there was more to life than a crazy family that was constantly morphing into something else. I was just a tween but had secretly started smoking and made friends who showed me how to sneak alcohol from the liquor cabinet without anybody knowing. My friend Stephanie taught me how to wear mascara and eyeliner, and I added tops that showed my midriff and big silver hoop earrings to my look. I padded my bra to make it look like I had breasts, even though I hadn't yet had my first period. I looked more like sixteen than twelve. And I was angry. I challenged my mother's rules and rebelled against everything that was expected of me. For entertainment, I went to big department stores and shoplifted makeup, and clothes, and underwear, and stuffed animals, and key chains. Things I didn't need. I did it for the thrill and never got caught—but I did have to run from a store security guard once. It just felt like icing on the cake. My friends were my accomplices. They were hesitant and nervous. I was ballsy and cocky, always going for bigger, pricier items or the things closest to the register. In short order, I had gone from a quiet, proper, straight-A student to a rebel who was always seeking out drama.

As much as I fought it, I had no choice but to surrender to the move to Lidingö. That meant a new school, of course. I didn't want to admit it but I desperately wanted to fit in and make friends, so I made my dad buy me a new pair of Diesel jeans. Lidingö was all about designer labels, fancy purses, and money and I had no idea how I would survive. All I knew was city life—I listened to hip-hop, smoked cigarettes, and spoke suburban slang.

The first day of high school was awful. I wore my new jeans and a trucker hat pulled down low, trying to keep my head down. In the hallway, a senior yelled at me, "It's okay to be a lesbian!" I thought I was going to sink through the floor and die. I looked like a lesbian? Was that a bad thing? I guessed yes. Was it my Diesel jeans? My hat? I had thought my hat was cool; it was what all my friends in the inner city wore. I took the hat off and stuffed it into my bag. I didn't speak to anyone all day and when I got home I cried to my mom, "It's *horrible*. I won't survive a week!" "Don't worry," she said. "You'll make friends." I scoffed and ran to my room, slamming the door behind me.

A day later, I came home with a new group of girlfriends. I'd hit it off with a girl in my class who was also a smoker (cigarettes, like broken bones, were good icebreakers) and had introduced me to her girl gang. My new friends were different from the ones I'd had in the inner city. Everyone had money, and it turned out—so did I! My father had become a nice source of revenue for new clothes, a brand-new scooter (so I could get to and from school without having to take the bus), and vacations with friends to places like the French Alps and the south of Spain. I'd never cared about money before—actually, I'd always been embarrassed about the fact that my dad was well-off—but now, living in one of the wealthiest areas of Stockholm, it was suddenly an asset.

One of those trips was to Åre, a ski resort in the north of Sweden. Some of the kids rented their own cabins and I was amazed at what they were allowed to do on their own at only fifteen years old. My dad had a vacation house in Åre so I stayed with him. I spent every night before my one o'clock curfew getting hammered on beer the bartenders snuck to us.

It was one of those nights at the bar I met Jonathan. He was tall and handsome, and the moment I saw him I felt butterflies in my stomach. There was something about him—he felt a little bit dangerous, and I liked it. The bonus was that he was four and a half years older and a good kisser. When the week in Åre ended and it was time for me to go home, he texted me. Want to hang out in Stockholm, too? Thus began what would turn into my first big love.

Something happened when Jonathan and I were together. It was like we were meant to be, like all the stars of the universe had aligned just to put us in each other's arms. When I was with him I didn't feel insecure anymore. I felt safe, at home. We started spending every waking second together and soon we seemed to disappear into each other.

Jonathan was a sweet guy but had a very troubled life. He made most of his money in less-than-legal ways, roped into criminal activity by his family. He told me he wanted to go to law school but that transitioning from easy money to a regular job was too difficult. He was also a graffiti artist and we spent most weekends driving around the city looking for the next canvas. I was on the lookout for cops while he and his friends painted huge murals across subway stations and tunnels. I loved it—the thrill of doing something dangerous excited me. Jonathan was insanely jealous, and over time, I became jealous, too. We'd go from intense lovemaking to screaming and throwing things at each other. When he got angry his eyes went black. The fighting was always followed by enormous passion, tears, and clinging tighter to each other than ever before. More than once he got into a bar fight over some guy looking at me. I liked that I had a man who would fight for me, but even at that young age a part of me wondered, *Is it supposed to be this hard?* Over time, his temper became my new normal, and when he chased me up the stairs to our house after a huge fight one evening and broke the window to my bedroom with his fist to grab me by the hair, I still didn't think he'd gone too far. Neither did I think so when—after a dinner party where I was seated next to a friend of his and I accused him of being delusional when he grew suspicious— he slapped me in the face under a streetlight and ripped my dress to shreds. Nor that one night he maced me in the face and I felt like I was going to suffocate. I thought it was love. In a strange way, it was.

During my senior year, I ditched my classes as often as I could to be with Jonathan. On my eighteenth birthday he gave me a ring and I accepted it. Eventually, we stopped leaving his apartment and would sleep until late in the afternoon. In the evenings, we drank. My life reeked of Bacardi Razz and cheap vodka. I had no clue what I wanted to do with my life, and even though I thought I'd found my soul mate, I was starting to feel really lost.

At the time, Mom was in the middle of divorcing Stefan Number Two and had recently spent a week at a meditation center looking for, and apparently finding, some answers. Knowing I was struggling, she recommended I go, too. A part of me was so terrified I thought I was literally going to die, but I went anyway. I was expecting to find the reasons behind my sadness, maybe work though some issues with my dad, but instead I found silence. The days were a mix of active meditations, group sessions, exercises for living a healthy life and, in between, absolute silence. It was in that silence I realized something momentous: I didn't have a clue as to who I was.

For as long as I could remember I hadn't been able to hear over the voice in my head that dictated my life. The voice that said I wasn't good enough, or pretty enough, or thin enough, or smart enough; the voice that said I didn't deserve love; that I deserved to have bad things happen to me; that life wasn't meant to be good and beautiful, only survived. As that voice began to quiet down, I started having profound realizations about my life. The many traumatic events from my childhood that had never healed resurfaced, everything from circumstances around my birth to my parents separating, my stepfather dying, moving from place to place, my mother's suicide attempt, my dad's absence, all the new family constellations, and the divorces that always followed . . . I saw that my life had been a series of separations and losses. How could I trust anyone or anything when I was always waiting for someone to leave me? I was eighteen and only just beginning to scratch the surface, but it was a start.

After a meditation on the last day it dawned on me that I had spent most of my life making decisions based off what would make other people happy. I'd been so confused, focusing on pleasing everyone but myself and bending over backward to try to fix the chaos around me. Sitting there on my meditation cushion, I realized: I don't want to go home. Immediately a twinge of guilt touched my heart—what would my mother say if I didn't come home? It would hurt her, surely. She would be upset. Having spent my whole life trying to avoid upsetting her, what objectively looked like an easy decision felt insurmountable. But . . . What did I feel? What about me? I picked up the notebook I'd been journaling in throughout the week. "What's the most loving thing to do?" I wrote in big letters across the page. We'd spent a lot of time at the center meditating on and talking about self-love, and how sometimes the most loving action to take isn't necessarily the easiest one. In that moment, everything became clear. Choosing to spare my mother's feelings by pretending everything was fine when it wasn't would not be a loving thing to do. Neither was ignoring my own needs to avoid confrontation, or choosing someone else's happiness over my own. "I choose myself," I wrote. "The most loving thing I can do, is to choose myself."

I left the retreat week with insight that I didn't know what to do with, and the realization that I was angry with my mom was a big one. It was a strange feeling. I'd never, ever been mad at her before. My main focus had always been keeping her happy and lifting her up, but I found that she was getting really heavy to carry. I knew I couldn't face her, feeling the way I did, and chose to stay with Jonathan instead of returning home when the retreat ended. I still thought of him as the only constant in my life, but when I saw him, I didn't feel the happiness I was expecting to feel. We made love the night I got back and I remember thinking, for the first time since we met, *I don't think this is it.* I had experienced such profound joy and release at the retreat center—why couldn't I hold on to that feeling when I was with him?

After that, I started making changes in my life. I quit smoking, *just like that.* I cut down on alcohol. There was something better out there than makeup and boys and drinking. Most important, I continued the inquiries I had started during my week away. For the first time in my young life I asked myself questions: *Does this make me happy? Is this where I'm supposed to be?* Life was pulling me in two directions. A part of me wanted to go back to my old unconscious self, and a part of me wanted to explore the new way of life I'd just had a taste of.

After a few months of fits and starts I returned to the center for another week of self-realization. It was even more intense than the first time. This one was heavily focused on childhood. A week of deep dives into my past was exhausting and so much emotion was surfacing I hardly knew what to do with it all. One morning I was walking into the meditation hall, dragging my feet at the thought of yet another dynamic meditation. Dynamic meditation is a meditation that allows for emotional release, using the body as a gateway into the heart. By moving intensely, we are able to quiet the mind and make our way toward deep stillness. It's as challenging as it is amazing. As I walked into the room, I saw a woman on a yoga mat, moving her body from pose to pose. I stopped to watch her. How could something be that important and feel so good that she rose earlier than everyone else to do it? It seemed so sacred. I had never felt that way about anything. *I want that*, I thought.

During the days that followed I unearthed more about my past than I ever had before. Memories I'd repressed came flooding out, and I realized that the anger I'd felt toward my mom after the first retreat was just the tip of the iceberg. One specific exercise involved an emotionally charged guided meditation followed by an exploration of our relationship with our mothers. After that they handed out crayons for us to draw a life-sized picture of our moms. When they introduced the exercise I thought it sounded ridiculous. I had to draw a picture of my mom? Really? I hadn't done that since I was a little girl. A memory surfaced: me sitting at our old kitchen table drawing a picture of my family with crayon. In stick figure shapes I drew me, my little brother, Stefan, and Mom. The memory made me smile, and then filled me with sadness. Why hadn't I included my dad? Even as a child I was confused about my family. No wonder I had to sit here at some retreat center to figure everything out. I felt anger bubble up inside me and before I knew it, I was sketching my mom with wide, harsh strokes on the giant roll of paper on the floor in front of me. When I'd finished I almost laughed. I still drew like a child. I had given my mom shoulder-length, straw-colored hair, and she was wearing a blue, triangle-shaped dress. Her mouth was drawn in an upside down U; she was sad. Of course she was sad. For as long as I could remember, she had been sad. Looking at the picture I'd drawn, it didn't look funny to me anymore.

Someone helped me hang the picture up on the wall in front of me, and soon I heard the facilitator's voice on the speakers. "Feel your body in this moment. What are you feeling? What's moving in your heart? If your mother was here, what would you tell her?" I remained silent, not knowing what to say. My mind told me this was ridiculous; I was supposed to speak to a drawing as if I were talking to my mom? It wasn't until I touched my hands to my face that I realized I was crying. Ridiculous or not, I was channeling emotions that were very real. "Move your body," the facilitator urged us. "Use your voice! See what comes." I heard people around me begin to talk and soon the room was filled with emotion. Using the energy of other people to get me going, I gave it a try. "You are always sad," I told the picture of my mom hanging in front of me. "You are *always sad!*" My voice was growing stronger. "Even when other people think you're happy, I can tell that you're sad. It's exhausting trying to make you happy all the time. I don't want to do it anymore." Suddenly, the words came pouring out of me. "Actually, I *can't* make you happy! I can't do it! It's exhausting just to try. Also, you left me. You tried to kill yourself! What kind of a mother does that to her own kids?" I don't know how it happened, but I was shouting now. Everything I'd always wanted to tell her but had been too afraid to speak out loud, I was telling her now. What had started off as sadness was transforming into anger. "*Why can't you just be happy like a normal mom???*" I shouted. I had spent my whole life worrying more about her than I did myself and it wasn't until now that I realized that I actually had eighteen years of bottled-up anger and resentment inside of me. *"I am so sick of your emotions! You take up too much space! There is no space for me to feel anything when you are so sad all the time!"* Every word that came out of my mouth came both as news to me—I didn't know that I had been feeling this way—and as something I knew as absolute truth. I had spent my whole life playing small to make space for her. I was always waiting for the other shoe to drop. Always waiting for her to leave me again. As I shouted I began stomping my feet—I was so, so angry. Someone handed me a big pillow and before I knew it I had collapsed on the ground, punching my fists into it with all of my might.

Tears were streaming down my face and my nose was full of snot, but I didn't care. In my eighteen years on this earth I had never before experienced a true release of emotion. It was absolutely cathartic and once I had started, I felt like I could go on forever. Anger and love and fear and sadness came pouring out of me, all wrapped up as one. In the midst of it all, I spoke a sentence that brought me to a full stop. "It wasn't my fault." It surprised me enough to actually stop me in my tracks. *Where did that come from? What wasn't my fault?* I said it again. "It wasn't my fault. It wasn't my fault. It wasn't my fault." I repeated it like a mantra, and as I did, something I had kept hidden in the deepest, darkest corners of my soul rose to the surface.

A part of me had always felt responsible for Stefan's death. As a child, I'd been convinced that it was my fault that he died, and although as an adult I could objectively see that it wasn't, there was a little five-year-old girl inside of me that felt responsible. That pain, that guilt, had been there my entire life. Speaking the truth out loud now was like casting a magic spell, freeing me from blame and responsibility. "It wasn't my fault. It wasn't my fault. *It wasn't my fault.*" I was crying intensely now, curled up in a ball, shaking with grief. Every tear I hadn't allowed myself to shed when the plane crashed, I cried now. The pain I'd never let myself feel when my mother tried to kill herself, I felt now. I cried for my mom and the horrible things she'd had to endure. I cried for my brother, who was so young. I cried for my dad, who I'd never seen cry, not once. But most of all I cried for myself. For having to grow up so fast. For the trauma I'd lived through. For the weight I'd had to carry my whole life. For the pain I'd carried. For the love I'd lost. For the guilt I'd held that wasn't mine.

I don't know how long I laid there on the floor crying, but by the time I opened my eyes a new version of me looked out at the world. I felt a thousand pounds lighter. Something huge had shifted inside of me. I could stand taller, breathe a little easier. It was sad, and it was beautiful. When the session came to a close I walked out of the room exhausted, but with the hint of a smile on my lips. I felt free.

Healing these broken parts of my past completely changed my life. I left the retreat floating, and started seeing how the things I was dealing with would keep resurfacing for as long as it took for me to figure them out. By finding the tools to deal with my past I was able to shed heavy layers of pain and defenses that had weighed me down for as long as I could remember. Without knowing exactly how, happiness began to seep in. I started eating healthier and meditating every day. I found myself waking up feeling . . . happy. Just, happy. It was a strange feeling, and something I'd never experienced before. *What kind of life could I create for myself out of this space?* I thought. Soon, I realized I had to get away. I didn't know where, just that it had to be without Jonathan. The journey I needed to go on was far outside of my comfort zone, and with him next to me I'd be stifled from challenging myself.

Before I could give it too much thought, the universe stepped in. Two friends asked me to join them on a trip to Costa Rica. I didn't hesitate. I saved up as much money as I could and hoped it was enough for three months of hostel stays. I was terrified to go—I think a part of me knew that there would be no turning back. At the airport I almost changed my mind; the thought of leaving Jonathan behind felt impossible. I cried so hard I couldn't breathe. It felt like a loss, probably because it was. I remembered one of the key insights I'd had at the meditation center: If you're ever at a crossroads, ask yourself which choice is more loving. And then go do that. In this situation—what was more loving? Staying behind, or moving forward? I closed my eyes. In my heart I already knew. Forward we go.

3

PRACTICE

From the moment my feet touched the ground in Costa Rica I felt divinely guided. My panic over leaving Jonathan subsided, and I met people who shared my new view of life. I felt like a snake shedding its skin. For every day that passed, I was becoming lighter, leaving pieces of my past behind. During those first weeks in Costa Rica I was able to rid myself of the preconceived ideas I'd had about who I was "supposed" to be, and for the first time in my life I started to feel like myself. Turns out, without that heavy past weighing me down, I was a pretty remarkable person! I felt like a magnet, attracting beautiful experiences everywhere I went. In Sweden I was alone on my newfound spiritual journey; I had thoughts and ideas about life that didn't fit with anyone I knew. Here, I felt completely at home. The anxiety that had filled my body for most of my life vanished and suddenly I felt strong, present, purposeful. I started journaling and devoured spiritual books like never before. Every day I got up before sunrise to sit on the beach and meditate. First I repeated the meditation techniques I'd learned at the retreat center, but soon I had a full library of different kinds of techniques and meditations to use. I had a revelation: if I did these things every day; if I sought out peace, it was actually available to me. I wasn't going to find it at the bottom of a tequila bottle or on the couch watching TV. The life I wanted wasn't going to fall into my lap one day—I had to get out there and fight relentlessly for it. And what a magical insight it was, that life didn't have to be so difficult! My whole life I'd felt like I was treading water, fighting for my life. And now, here I was, my feet in the warm sand, no idea what the future would bring, and I felt more at peace than I ever had before. Who knew life could be this easy?

My friends and I swam in the ocean, ate locally grown foods, hiked through the rain forest, and danced all night. We stayed in hostels with scorpions and cockroaches, traveled on buses down dusty roads to explore the Pacific coast, and got so used to lugging our backpacks around they became like extra limbs. I felt like I had entered a whole new phase of life, with a brand-new version of myself. Every day I was growing more independent. Meditation became as easy as breathing. The world was my oyster and everything was new. I didn't want to cling to that old part of me that I'd been holding on to out of fear of the unknown. I started to trust myself.

Still, almost every day I made my way to a pay phone to call Jonathan. He was my one connection to my old life, and I felt the contrast with the life I was creating in Costa Rica. I started dreading going to the phone booth and began putting the calls off more and more. I still loved him, but talking to him felt like wearing shoes that were two sizes too small. I'd grown, and it seemed like the rest of my life back home hadn't caught up. During one of those calls, Jonathan said he'd gotten a tattoo of my name. I froze. A part of me already knew deep down that he wasn't my future, but I hadn't been able to figure out exactly how that would happen. He'd sensed I was drifting away . . . so he tattooed my name across his back. The permanence of a tattoo shook me into the reality that I wasn't in love with him anymore. This next chapter was about me, but the transition wasn't going to be easy. We'd been together for all of my adult life—I grew up alongside of him. And worst of all: I would have to break his heart. The thought of it pained me and I wasn't sure I'd be able to go through with it. Again, I had to ask myself: What is more loving? Is there a loving way to break someone's heart? I went to meditate at sunrise one morning and, holding my hands to my heart, I felt all the love I had for Jonathan. It was huge—but there was something in the way. I loved him, but I wasn't in love with him anymore. I was falling in love with myself! And that relationship wasn't something I was prepared to let go of—I'd just found it. Continuing down this path with Jonathan felt impossible. I didn't want to pretend or have to fake it—it would be an even bigger betrayal. Tears started streaming down my face as I realized the inevitable decision I'd arrived at: the most loving thing was to let go.

My friends and I made our way down to Dominical, a dusty little surf town south of where most tourists go. It was a quiet town, and we found a hostel a short walk from the beach. We took surf lessons, shopped handmade bracelets from vendors, and drank cold beer at sunset. I had barely had time to unpack my backpack when I met Mike, the manager of a vegan restaurant in town. Mike was tanned and muscular in that surfer way, with big brown eyes and an irresistible smile. I'd been with Jonathan for almost four years and never before felt the urge to be with someone else. And now here was this guy, the opposite of Jonathan—laid-back, easygoing, happy—and our attraction to each other was palpable.

Mike had left the States to move to Costa Rica and he was vegan and all about natural living. He woke up at sunrise every morning—just like me—to meditate and surf and was so excited about a new project he was working on: a way to transform his diesel engine to run on vegetable oil. Everything about him was new and intriguing. With him, I felt like I could be whoever I wanted to be. I didn't have to be Rachel with the sad story, or Rachel the party girl. I was just Rachel, the current, evolving version, the Rachel who meditated, who loved to read, who wanted to travel the world and discover all that life had to offer. I broke up with Jonathan by phone immediately, feeling so detached from my old life and so sure of what was ahead that it didn't hurt as much as I thought it would. I tried to keep the phone call as brief as I could, thinking it was best to just rip off the Band-Aid. The truth was, I didn't want to stick around long enough to hear the agony in his voice. I barely paused to think about the chaos I had created back home; I just wanted to be happy. *Jonathan would find a way to be happy on his own, too*, I thought.

A few weeks after we met, I spent the night with Mike. It was so different from anything I'd ever experienced. Lovemaking with Jonathan was passionate. With Mike it was soft, gentle, and easy. I started spending every night with him at his house in the jungle. I stopped wearing makeup and transitioned into veganism. I devoured every book on the subject I could find and soaked up knowledge like a sponge. I'd never given any thought to my diet before that—no one had told me about the meat industry and what excess animal protein does to your body. My new diet changed my body—my skin cleared up and the asthma I'd suffered since childhood subsided. After a while many of the allergies I'd struggled with for most of my life completely disappeared. Every day I felt better, stronger, and healthier. There was no stress in my body, no worries, no anxiety. I felt so at home, not just in Costa Rica but within myself.

After three months in paradise, it was time to go home. As the trip wound down, I knew one thing for sure: this was not the end of my journey—it was the beginning. Mike drove us all to the airport in San José, and although it was hard leaving him because we had fallen in love, it wasn't the end of the world. I knew I would see him again, but part of me knew he wasn't my end game either—just an important piece of my moving forward.

I landed in Sweden feeling like a brand-new version of myself. I was the healthiest I'd ever been, calm, confident, and happy. The first thing I found when I came home was a huge box on my bedroom floor with all the things I'd ever given Jonathan. Our whole lives were there—most of it smashed to pieces or shredded. I sat down, and looking through the things—photographs, birthday gifts, paintings he'd made me—I felt like I was looking at someone else's life. I didn't regret breaking up with him. It was what had to be done. Mike and I stayed in touch, and a few months later, he traveled to Sweden to see me. I was still enchanted by him, but my inner voice was telling me this wasn't it. However, detaching has never been my strong suit. Having Mike in Sweden was great, but we didn't have the same easygoing flow that we did in Costa Rica. Almost immediately, I started noticing him distancing himself from me: he slept with his back to me, and he wouldn't hold my hand in public. I felt starved for attention. I wanted Mike to be "the one" so badly that I ignored the signs he wasn't. Instead, I focused on superficial things to place distance between us; for instance, the baggy jeans he wore that I thought were so sexy in the jungle were all of a sudden the wrong fit and made him look sloppy. In Costa Rica he was the perfect man. In Sweden, things didn't feel right anymore, but that didn't stop me from pretending.

At my dad's invitation, we traveled from Sweden to Spain. It was a beautiful week of eating tapas, walks along the beach, and shopping in the little markets scattered around town. The weird feelings I had in Sweden let up and by the end of the week when it was time for Mike to fly back to Costa Rica, I was sad to see him go. My dad was leaving for Sweden that same day and I decided to stay in Spain on my own for a little while. I didn't know what I wanted to do in life—where did I belong? I needed alone time to figure it out. When everyone was gone, I felt empty, hollow, and drained. I couldn't figure out why I was suddenly so unhappy.

After crying all the tears I'd bottled up inside, I drew myself a bath, added some lavender oil, and laid down in the hot water. Slowly, I felt my body relaxing and my breath returning. *Okay*, I told myself, *so I'm alone now. I can be alone. I can be independent.* I realized that it wasn't until I was alone that I started feeling like myself again. I had a pattern when it came to relationships, where I was so scared of being abandoned that I'd fully change who I was to try to fit in with the other person. It had been exhausting, spending those weeks with Mike. I didn't know it until just now, but I'd actually been longing to be alone. I remembered: my most important relationship is with myself. In the blink of an eye I stopped feeling sad and decided to focus on the art of being by myself.

The next morning I got up at sunrise and sat down on the patio to meditate. After a few deep breaths I felt all the tension draining from my body. I hadn't meditated a single time since arriving in Europe. Now, finally sitting in silence again, I felt myself grounding. When I finished my session, a memory came to me. I was transported back into the meditation hall at the retreat center the year before, where I saw the woman stretching on her yoga mat, having woken up before everyone else to practice. I decided I could move my body like that, too. I normally suffered from a lot of back pain, but it had eased up a lot over the past few months. I stood up and started to stretch. I wasn't aware of what a yoga practice entailed, or if I was doing real yoga poses, but the thought of being alone on a yoga mat—like the woman I had seen at the retreat—was what I wanted to connect to. All I knew was, it felt good!

After breakfast I headed down to the harbor and went to the bookstore. The first thing that caught my eye was a book about yoga. I bought it, and in the spur of the moment headed into a sport shop next door and picked up a yoga mat as well. As soon as I got home I started reading the book; when evening came, I rolled out my brand-new mat and sat in meditation. Just as it had that morning, something about the silence of meditation made me yearn to move and stretch. Using the book as my guide, I made my way into a reclined twist. I lay down, crossed my legs, and dropped them over to one side. I heard my back crackle and pop. It surprised me but actually felt good. I moved to the other side, and then continued through a few more poses from the book. Downward-Facing Dog was a challenge—my wrists hurt and the backs of my legs burned. But after a few poses I started getting the hang of it and realized that, just like with medi-tation, if I stayed connected to my breath and brought my attention inward, it was easy. At the end I laid down in some-thing the book called Savasana—just lying flat on my back on the floor. Closing my eyes, I felt a sense of calm wash over me. I don't know how long I laid there, but when I opened my eyes the stars had come out. *Wow*, I thought. *This yoga thing might just be something.*

Newly inspired, I went back to the bookstore for books about crystals, meditation, and veganism. I started cooking everything from scratch and experimented with new foods and flavors. I discovered I could cook! I'd never cooked in my life, but now I felt a passion for food. Every day I rolled out my yoga mat on the patio, meditated, and practiced yoga. In the evenings I spent hours in the kitchen cooking elaborate meals for myself. My European solo vacation became about meditation, yoga, and cooking vegan food.

I ended up staying in Spain for more than a month. Most of the time I felt at peace, but I still suffered moments of anxiety—always related to Mike. Every time Mike didn't respond fast enough to an e-mail, or call when I thought he should, I felt abandoned. I became obsessive about making sure we spoke every day, and the more I forced it, the more I felt him pull away. Negative thoughts swirled in my head. *What if he doesn't love me? . . . Why isn't he calling more? . . . Maybe I'm not good enough.* It was the first time I was faced with the disparity between my ability to be present and my mind's constant attraction to worst-case scenarios. I was reading *The Power of Now* by Eckhart Tolle and started to think that maybe my obsessive negative thoughts weren't true. If I could stay in the moment and just be, I'd always come back to the same conclusion: all is well. Every time my mind took control, I challenged myself not to get pulled into panic mode. It became a routine: feeling calm and independent and grounded, and at some point being catapulted into anxiety by something as simple as Mike not returning a phone call.

I realized that this was a practice: I was reconditioning my mind, and to do that, I needed challenges like these. The codependency issues I shared with Jonathan hadn't simply gone away when he did. They were still there. But now I was in a relationship with a guy who wasn't in that same space, a guy who was used to living on his own, doing his own thing, and having casual relationships. In Costa Rica I had been this confident, breezy girl, but the more serious the relationship got, the more the old me forced her way back and I'd become needy—almost desperate—for love and attention. Of course Mike was pulling away. I asked myself relevant questions: Did I actually love Mike? Did my relationship with him mirror the new, evolved me? Or had I just been fooling him—and myself—when I'd presented myself the way I had at the beginning? Was Mike my forever guy, or a transition from my old life to the one in which I was headed? I spent weeks pondering these questions, journaling, meditating, shifting between struggle and ease. Practicing.

On my last night in Spain I went down to the water and sat at a little bar perched right in the sand. I ordered a glass of white wine, something I normally wouldn't do. It felt like a very grown-up thing to do: sit alone at sunset with a glass of wine. I was only nineteen and there was so much I'd never done on my own. I'd had a ton of alcohol in my life, but always with the intention to disappear into it, to forget, or to escape. Drinking that crisp glass of wine, I realized that the alcohol wasn't the problem—it was a symptom. I could make everything excessive and turn anything into a problem, just as I could make anything sacred if I did it with consciousness and presence. Watching the sky turn to pink and purple and gold, I wrote in my journal. I had done so much growing since I'd been there, and most important, I'd been completely on my own. I felt a calm within me now that wasn't as easily shaken by outside events, and I was beginning to understand that there was a greater purpose to the challenges thrown my way.

As I drank my wine, with my feet snugly in the sand, a smile spread across my face. I wrote: "This is a perfect moment." It was. I was just beginning to grasp that the love I'd been seeking so desperately in others was really within myself.

I returned to Stockholm ready to figure out my next move. On a whim, I visited my friends Olivia and Daniella in my old hometown of Uppsala and ended up signing up for classes at the university there. It was a spur-of-the-moment thing—I didn't know what I wanted to do next so why not study for a semester? I planned to return to Costa Rica, but it wasn't about Mike. Going back had to be about me. I needed my own purpose, my own reason, to stay on my own path. I knew I had to save up some money to be able to go and not look back, so I decided to tend bar at a restaurant in town. I studied by day and my nights were spent serving up twenty-dollar drinks.

I'd been talking to Mike less and less and one day he called to say he'd met someone else. I was sad, but glad he was man enough to be truthful. Holding on to a piece of him, even from afar, meant I wasn't completely on my own and now I really was. Rather than scare me, the realization filled me with a sense of empowerment. I had my entire life ahead of me—I could do whatever I wanted to do. The thought was exhilarating.

One semester was enough time for me to realize that university life wasn't for me. By then I had saved enough tip money to return to Costa Rica. It was only a question of when I'd go. The answer fell out of the sky one morning when I woke up. My feet ached from working a double shift the night before. It was freezing outside, the coldest winter in thirty years, and I dreaded getting out of bed. As I looked out at the gray sky, something inside of me clicked. *Yes. It's time*, I thought. That same day I booked a one-way ticket to Costa Rica. I had to spend that time back in Sweden to fully arrive at my own conclusion: I wasn't supposed to do this the way all of my friends did. University wasn't for me. Sweden wasn't either. I belonged by the ocean.

4
___

FORGIVE

Being back in Costa Rica felt like coming home. I got on the bus at the airport and headed straight for Dominical. I was a little bit nervous, not knowing what to expect, arriving completely alone. I had a few friends in town, but things were different this time around; I was on my own. I checked into a hostel with the plan to find a permanent place to stay as soon as possible.

Settling back into life there was easier than I'd anticipated. I got a job as a server at an Italian restaurant in town and started bartending at two different bars. I didn't have a big-picture plan. I just wanted to make enough money to get by. I wanted to swim in the ocean every day. I wanted to feel free. In my spare time I practiced yoga, lounged in a hammock at the local dive shop, and hung out with the tourists. The manager of the dive shop was a girl named Laura whose husband was a dive master. I hadn't really made any close girlfriends during my previous stay. Making friends with women didn't come naturally to me; I'd always felt more at ease with men. My friendship with Laura happened pretty much by default. She told me she didn't like me at first. I was "too loud, too blond, and too tall," she said. I guess I wore her down, because eventually we struck up a friendship.

Laura practiced yoga at a small studio in town and I started tagging along. At the same time, I continued what I'd started in Spain—devouring spiritual books and teachings, eager to deepen both my meditation and yoga practice. I felt more empowered and more at peace than I ever had. I was finally living on my own and making choices for me with nothing to hold me back! Because I felt at peace, I created it everywhere I went. The strangest things happened; I would think of something and it magically manifested. I sat on the beach, longing for a coconut, and a friend suddenly walked by and offered me one. Whenever I needed extra money, a customer at the restaurant would give me a huge tip. Things like that. After a few months I began taking my newfound ability for granted. I got to a place where I could listen to my iPod, put all thousand-plus songs on shuffle, and know which song would play next. Now I know it as the law of attraction—your thoughts become your reality—but at the time it seemed more like magic.

After working at the restaurant for what felt like too long, I was ready for something more adventurous, and right on cue, an opportunity presented itself. I was chatting with a table of customers one day, and before they paid the bill, I had a new job. Their company was in the process of acquiring land to build sustainable hotels. I was hired as the personal assistant to the head of the initiative, a man named John. It was a new position, and I think neither John nor I had any idea what it would entail. He told me he'd felt so strongly about having me on the team that he created the position for me. I did everything from administrative and e-mail work to more personal things like booking travel and keeping the team healthy with vegetarian food and fresh smoothies every day. One morning during a break, I rolled my mat out on the patio of the house the company was working from. I practiced the poses the way I'd learned them, feeling so comfortable in each one by now that they came without my having to think about what to do. When I walked back to the house John stopped me. "Can you teach us that?" he asked. "Teach you what?" I asked. "Yoga. It would be a nice thing for the team to do together in the mornings." I thought about it. Teach yoga? Me? "Sure," I said. "Absolutely." The next day I guided John through a series of postures, speaking while I moved. I didn't have to pause and think about what I was doing, even though I'd never taught it before. Strangely, it flowed naturally. At the end of the session a thought hit me. *Had I just taught my first yoga class?*

One of the main properties the company was involved with was owned by a family who had started a commune, an intentional community, years before. I'd never seen anything like that—a group of thirty-some people, living together by choice in the rain forest. They shared chores—everything from tending to the grounds to cooking and cleaning. There was a strong spiritual component; everyone meditated and many practiced yoga, and they spoke to one another in a frank and honest way. Everyone had a say in how the property was used, so we spent a lot of time there and engaged in a lot of intense discussions—

usually about communal finances. When long days turned to night, I joined in the meditation circles.

One day John told me the commune was hosting a cacao shaman at the farm and that there would be a chocolate ceremony later in the day. I had heard of chocolate ceremonies for emotional healing and I was intrigued. A cacao shaman works with special types of beans from sacred parts of South America. An ancient ritual to prepare the cacao involves roasting and grinding the beans, then mixing the hot chocolate with brown sugar or agave syrup and cayenne pepper in a large pot. Cacao increases the blood flow to the heart and frees the heart chakra. Emotionally it translates to releasing pent-up feelings, and the ritual can be both intense and therapeutic.

John and I arrived at the farm in the early afternoon and joined the group on the patio. The circle of twenty or so people, some of them new faces, sat around the big pot of bubbling cacao. I'd never met a shaman before and was intrigued to see what he would look like. I envisioned an indigenous man, dressed in beads and robes. Instead, I arrived to find that the shaman was an American man in his sixties, with white hair and a long white beard. I sat down in the circle feeling a little wary—what had I signed up for? Of all places, the shaman sat down right next to me and we locked eyes. Looking into his clear, blue eyes, I felt a jolt of electricity zap through my body. It felt as if he were looking into the depths of my soul.

"Interesting," he said. "We're going to do you last." I had no idea what he meant, but I felt chills up and down my spine. We all drank the cacao and my mouth went dry from its bitter, spicy taste. This tasted nothing like the hot cocoa I used to drink on ski trips back home! My friends from the farm told me it could take some time for the cacao to "work its magic," but it was only a few minutes before I felt myself welling up with emotion. How did I end up here? In the middle of the jungle, with people I barely knew but somehow trusted deeply? The circle felt absolutely sacred, filled with a golden glow.

One of the attendees was a sweet man named Jesse who lived on the farm and had come to the ceremony with his wife and kids. Jesse was a realtor in town and a friend of John's. His last name was Angell (seriously!). I felt curiously drawn to his four-year-old daughter, Grace, who sat on a cushion—cross-legged, eyes closed, fingers in a gyan mudra—meditating. Grace wasn't trying to be present the way the others were. She just was. Seeing her so intensely present without effort awakened something deep inside of me. We were all just trying to make our way back to what we already are! We are born this way, full of light, emanating love. We see it in children; it's effortless. But somehow we get lost along the way. I felt a light emanate from Grace straight into my heart and, before I knew it, I had lost track of time and space. My eyes were open but I was breathing so deeply, completely immersed in the intricate workings of the moment unfolding around me. I felt one with the circle, one with the earth and the sky, one with all, and it lasted for what felt like forever. It was the most intense spiritual experience I had ever had. There was no thought, no ego, just light.

Meanwhile, the shaman worked his way around the circle, taking his time with each person, sitting with them, guiding them deeper. Eventually, after many hours, I was the only one left. Turning to me, he spoke out loud to the whole group. "We are about to enter a very sacred space together now." I heard his voice clearly, but it was as if I were somewhere else. I felt like I was floating above the ground. "You are on the verge of something life changing," he told me. "Everyone has a purpose in life, but it's very rare that I meet someone and immediately know theirs. I knew it the moment I looked into your eyes. And you are meant to realize and understand it now, too." When he said this, I started crying, but it was different from the tears I had shed in the past. I wasn't gasping for breath or wiping snot from my nose. Streams of tears flowed, no, poured from my eyes, but it didn't feel like I was crying. It felt like I was purging. *These are not my tears*, I thought. But if they weren't mine, where were they coming from? "They're your ancestors' tears," the shaman said, as if he'd heard my thoughts. "That light you're feeling in your chest? We all feel it, too. Keep expanding it. Keep breathing into it. We are going to move into your ancestry now. It's a dark place and you're going to need to bring this light with you."

I did as he said and closed my eyes. "Standing behind you are your ancestors," the shaman said. "To your left is your mother. To your right is your father." Behind them were their parents—my grandparents—and behind them theirs, and so on, he said, "creating an infinite triangle of generations behind you and forming the entirety of your past and your lineage. As you can feel, your ancestry is weighed heavy with pain."

Suddenly, I was overcome with emotion. I still felt the light emanating from my chest, but the rest of my body grew heavy with sadness and fear. Visions came before my eyes that felt like memories. I saw it all so clearly. Just like the tears I was crying weren't mine, the memories I saw flash in front of my eyes weren't mine either. I saw my dad, as an infant, being thrown across the room by his father in a fit of rage; whipped with a belt; abandoned in a sterile hospital bed. My mother as a little girl with bruises on her arms, all alone and crying under her bedcovers while her sisters ate dinner with my grandmother in another room. My grandmother as a child locked in a cold dirt basement, the space so small she couldn't stand up or lie down. My grandfather, chased down by his dad and beaten with a closed fist. The flashes of abuse went so far back that I didn't recognize the children in them anymore, but I felt their fear and their sadness intensely. I was witnessing abusive behavior as it was passed down through generations. I felt my whole being weighed down with pain and sadness, but if I kept breathing into the light in my heart the way the shaman guided me to, it was bearable. Vision after vision passed in front of my eyes, and although I wasn't speaking, the shaman was able to address them all. He saw what I saw. After a while, I felt myself strangely distant from yet intricately connected to what I was seeing. A part of me understood: this all lives in me. I was witnessing pain passed down from person to person, and however awful it was, it was what it was. I couldn't change it. It was the past I'd been given, and it was given to me for a reason. In an instant I had a massive revelation: None of the people in my family had acted with intentional cruelty. They were acting out what they knew, repeating a pattern that started long before their own consciousness, generations before they were even born. The trauma was passed on to them and, strangely, they had no other choice. This was the best they could do.

Finally, I saw myself as a child, and all of the emotional damage that was done to me. I saw glimpses of my mother's depression, her suicide attempt, leaving me alone to take care of myself. All the separation and divorce in our family. I saw my father abandoning us to start another family. Threatening us. Yelling at me. With every flashback I felt the pain I'd been carrying for so many years. With that came the insight that I'd lived my life up to that point with the idea that my parents "should" have done things differently—as if they had made a conscious decision to bring about such hurt. Once I could see and feel what they endured as children, my own childhood began to make more sense. In one swift moment, I understood that my parents loved me the only way they knew how. They had done the best with what they were given. What more could I possibly ask?

The next breath I took was so deep it felt like the whole of the universe was breathing through me. As I breathed out, I exhaled much of the resentment I'd been carrying for most of my adult life. The pain was still there, but it was bearable now. There was still healing left to do, but the weight of my sadness was lighter. With that realization, I cried so hard it felt as if the world was crying through me. I'd been right earlier when I'd thought my tears were not mine. They were the tears of an entire lineage, of all of my ancestors combined. I cried for my mother, for my father, who were just children once, too. I cried for my grandparents and for their parents. I cried for every child who had ever felt unsafe, for every moment of pain they'd ever endured. I cried for all of humanity until, suddenly, there were no tears left to cry.

When I opened my eyes again, it was getting dark outside. The whole day had passed and the only people remaining were the shaman, my boss, John, and a woman I didn't know. They were all looking at me with tears rolling down their cheeks. The shaman spoke to me: "It is your life's purpose to take on the accumulated pain of your ancestors, carry it on your shoulders, and transform it to light throughout your lifetime." As he was speaking, I felt a palpable light shining from my chest. If light was a feeling, this was it. "This all ends with you. All of this pain—it ends here. It's a heavy life purpose to have, but you can do it. It's why you are here. This pain ends with you. Your daughter will be the first in your lineage not to take it on." Goose bumps suddenly covered my body. "My daughter?" I asked. "Yes," he replied. "Your daughter. Spirit has great plans for her, too." I smiled. One day. A daughter. Looking at the others, he said, "Place your hands on Rachel. She needs to feel this connection." They did as they were told, but I felt uncomfortable. My own hands were on fire—I didn't need people to put their hands on me. I needed to put my hands on someone else. I turned around and put my hands on John's and the woman's backs. It felt like flames were shooting out of my palms. John later said it felt like he was being lifted off the ground.

I don't know how long we sat there, the four of us, on that wooden deck, but I felt the need to rest, so I closed my eyes. When I awakened, I was alone. A quiet rain fell on the tin roof, and a mist rose from the grass. The light I'd felt emanating from my body earlier was still there, and my heart felt like it was swelling out of my chest. Everything was so unbearably beautiful. The silence was otherworldly, like nothing I'd ever experienced. But it wasn't that the world had gone quiet. It was my mind. The incessant chatter I'd lived with, that little voice in the back of my head that said, *You're not good enough . . . no one loves you . . . that's why everyone abandons you*—the voice I was only ever able to quiet during moments of intense meditation—that voice was quiet. The silence was coming from within. *Is this enlightenment?* I wondered. With that thought came the instant realization that it wasn't, because if it were, I wouldn't be asking the question. I felt no disappointment. Okay, it wasn't enlightenment. But it was damn close.

I stood up; my pink and turquoise dress was sticky with sweat. Stretching my arms above my head, I let out a deep sigh. With my mind still quiet I stepped barefoot out into the jungle. I felt reborn. I walked into the woods. Everything was shining, as if dusted with glittering light. I walked for a bit and then laid down, belly first, with my face buried in the wet grass. I inhaled the earth and felt at one with it—the soil, the trees, every blade of grass. Soon, a deeper knowing sunk in: I am this earth. This earth is me. Everything is alive, like I am. We are alive together. All those clichés I'd heard in yoga class, or in meditation circles, or read in spiritual books were true. We are one.

By the time I got back to the farm the sun had set. I stepped onto the deck where the ceremony had been held, still feeling the vibration of the deep healing that had taken place. I longed for my mother and father. I yearned to tell them how much I loved them. "That was a wild ride!" someone said. I turned around. The shaman. "Yes," I said. "It was—" He interrupted me. "No need to explain," he said. "Stay silent, let it integrate. What you did here today was life changing. Healing moves both ways. Old generations and new. You have a great, big purpose in life. Don't lose sight of it." After a moment he asked, "Have you recently been invited to an ayahuasca ceremony?"

How did he know? A week earlier I'd been invited to an ayahuasca retreat but, after much contemplation, decided to decline. Ayahuasca is a vine with hallucinogenic properties that is boiled into a tea and used for intense spiritual awakening. I was a little overwhelmed by the idea. "Normally I recommend against it," the shaman said. "You see, with cacao, you take it on your own journey. You are only faced with what you are ready for. You steer the ship. But ayahuasca . . . it takes you on its *own* ride—you have no control. It can be a scary thing, taking the medicine. But I feel intensely that you have been called to do it. If you have the opportunity, go."

Putting his hand on my shoulder, he smiled. "Remember: there is nothing to fear," he said, his eyes twinkling. "There is only love."

5

SURRENDER

A day later, John called me to say he had decided to attend an ayahuasca ceremony and he thought I should come, too. Everything is divine, I thought. Nothing is random. I hadn't told him that the shaman already urged me to take part.

A girl named Kim from the farm joined John and me, and I brought my new puppy, Quila. Kim was familiar with ayahuasca and told us what to expect. The medicine would show us what we were avoiding and force us to deal with painful things from our past, she said. The purpose was to clear out negativity and old wounds for optimal spiritual healing. "But it's a hallucinogenic, isn't it?" I asked. I'd never been into drugs of any kind. I'd done my fair share of experimentation as a teenager but nothing I wanted to repeat. I didn't even smoke weed, unlike almost everyone else I knew. I didn't like losing control, and every time I'd tried it, marijuana left me feeling uneasy. Ayahuasca wasn't technically a drug but a deeply spiritual ritual, an ancient ceremony performed by indigenous shamans in certain parts of the world. Yes, the substance used was a hallucinogenic, Kim said. "But nothing like mushrooms or LSD." I had no experience with either mushrooms or LSD so I didn't quite understand what that meant. I decided to trust that I was put on this path for a reason, but I was still afraid.

The retreat center was in a remote location with no easy way to get there. We drove for hours to get to the nearest town, then navigated a small boat through the mangroves and arrived at a deserted beach just as the sun was setting. I saw, in the distance, a small figure dressed in bright pink. As we got closer, I could see it was a man who was very small and very old, wearing indigenous clothing and white face paint. He was smiling, his hands joined at the center of his chest in prayer. Now this was what I'd envisioned a shaman to look like! But I knew now, light comes in any form. In the cacao ceremony, it was four-year-old Grace who had initiated me. In a way, she was a shaman, too.

The man gestured for us to follow him into the jungle. He was barefoot but maneuvered the narrow paths like a child, jumping across rocks and balancing on roots sticking out of the ground. After a bit of a hike we got to the retreat center. It was bathed in candlelight, and a group of twenty or so people were gathered around a table, talking. They were stunned by the fact that we were there—there was no electricity at the center, and since we had decided to join in several days into the retreat, no one knew we were coming. They had all been eating dinner when the shaman suddenly stood up and announced, "They are here," and left the table. How did he know we were coming? I was in awe. This shaman . . . it was the real deal.

He only spoke the indigenous language of his tribe and had an interpreter there from their village, translating in Spanish. When I asked how old he was, he smiled and spoke in a tongue I didn't recognize. "He says he's not sure," the interpreter said. "He thinks, a hundred and twenty-seven." I smiled, as if he were joking, but his face was serious. They gave us small huts for sleeping, and we prepared for the big ayahuasca ceremony that was to take place the following day.

The next morning I practiced yoga on a big deck overlooking the rain forest. Kim was a Kundalini teacher and she guided me through some deeper breath work. We spent the day walking the grounds and hiking to the ocean for a swim, waiting for sunset for the ceremony to begin.

With the sun low on the horizon, I dressed in white, increasingly nervous as the time approached. By then I'd learned more about what was ahead: The ayahuasca vine, the plant itself, is boiled in water for several days until it reduces to a thick, syrupy substance. The "tea" is potent and very powerful. Some of the participants shared stories of visiting other dimensions, or horror-like visions and nightmarish experiences after they took it. The idea was to move through the fear to light and freedom. I remembered what the chocolate shaman told me: There is nothing to fear. There is only love.

At sunset, I walked to a huge open-air space where the ceremony was to take place. Hammocks hung from the wooden ceiling, which I thought was strange. The man who had translated for me the night before introduced himself as Rodrigo, the shaman's interpreter and our guide. "You are Raquel, yes?" he asked in Spanish. I often introduced myself as Raquel when I spoke Spanish. "This will be your hammock," he said, pointing to a blue and green hammock hanging from a wooden beam. "No, that's okay," I said. I was fluent in Spanish and grateful for my time immersed in the language. I politely declined. "I don't need a hammock. I like to move around." I had envisioned myself drinking the ayahuasca tea and being overcome with movement and spirit, dancing around the room. "No, amor." Rodrigo smiled, but I couldn't read his expression. "No vas a mover. La medicina, te paraliza," he said. "Te paraliza??" I said. Did I understand him correctly? The medicine would paralyze me?

I felt a tightening of my chest. *Ayahuasca paralyzes you? I'm going to willingly drink a tea that will turn me into a vegetable?* I panicked. Leaving Rodrigo midsentence, I ran from the deck out onto a path leading toward the jungle. After a few minutes I found a log and sat down. *What had I gotten myself into?* My chest was heaving. As I looked up at a golden sky I heard a voice say, "*Trust!*" It was stern and came from deep within my chest. The hair on my arms stood up. *How could I possibly trust when I was so fearful?* I wondered. Well, I hadn't traveled this far just to turn around and leave. I decided the only way to find out was to dive in.

Back on the deck, others were starting to gather. In the middle of the space was a huge firepit along with crystals, sage, and a big pot containing what I assumed was the medicine. Pitchers of water with ylang-ylang flowers sat nearby. The shaman was already seated, with his eyes closed and his head bowed. When Rodrigo saw me he took my hand. "Trust," he said. My eyes widened. "Trust that you are here for a reason."

Hearing him repeat the very same word that had just brought me back from panic calmed me completely. He guided me to my hammock. "If at any point during the night you need anything whatsoever—support, help, or if you need to throw up, anything at all—just call my name," he said. "I'll be by your side the entire time." Other participants had told me about the purging ayahuasca induced; it was common to vomit. The ceremony was to last from sundown to sunrise.

The air was electric and everyone seemed riveted. I was about to step into my hammock when Kim walked over. "I have something for you," she said, handing me a string of pale pink crystals. "Listen. There will be a point during the night when you will be certain you are going to die," she said. "You can't escape it. When that happens, move into Child's Pose and pray. Pray to God, to the Universe, to Great Spirit—pray to everything you believe in. Keep the crystals with you. They'll help. Ask for divine guidance. Ask God to save you." I was terrified. At one point I am going to be certain I'm going to die? *What am I getting myself into?* Kim rubbed lavender oil on my wrists. "The crystals and the oil will help you," she said. "Just trust." There was that word again. I closed my eyes and held on to the crystals. Taking a deep breath, I climbed into the hammock.

The shaman began chanting and drumming. There were a few more than twenty of us, each person suspended in a hammock hanging from the ceiling. The drumming intensified, and my breath became slow and steady. For what felt like a long time, I lay back in the hammock and watched the sky turn a golden, fiery orange. The drums, the smell of smoke from the fire, and the shaman's chant were all so mesmerizing, I felt like I was in a daze. I don't know how much time had passed but it was dark out when Rodrigo finally guided me to the fire. I took a seat in front of the shaman. He was seated on the ground, eyes closed, chanting feverishly. Someone holding a giant bundle of burning sage spoke in a language I didn't recognize. The shaman spat and gurgled as his chants grew louder. Abruptly, he stopped. He opened his eyes and looked at me. I could hear my heartbeat in my ears. He gave me a nod, then took a wooden ladle and stirred the pot. *Ayahuasca. The medicine*. He spooned some into a coconut shell and handed it to me. It was brownish black and as thick as molasses. He nodded as if to say "Go on." I gulped down the brew. It was so bitter I had to fight the urge to spit it right out. Rodrigo handed me a glass of ylang-ylang water. "Don't swallow it. It's just to clean the mouth," he said. I took a healthy swig, swirled it around in my mouth, and spat it out. *What now?* I wondered. Rodrigo guided me back to my hammock and I climbed in. They had told me it would take several hours for the effects to kick in, but just as with the cacao, I felt something move inside of me almost immediately.

At first I couldn't pinpoint what was happening, except that I started feeling overwhelmed. I tried to relax and focus on my breathing, but something inside of me was moving, and not in a good way. The breeze moving through the trees that was so gentle and soothing just a second ago started sounding like a thunderstorm. The rhythmic beat of the drums that I'd enjoyed moments earlier made me feel tense. I heard what sounded like killer waves crashing all around me. *The ayahuasca*, I thought. *It's working.*

The sounds around me grew louder and louder. The sound of the ocean, which I knew was a far trek away, became so loud I thought my eardrums might burst. I covered my ears, trying to block out the noise. The heat from the lavender oil that Kim had rubbed on my wrists started burning my skin. The air seemed to be frying my face. Everything became so intense so quickly and I realized: this is going to be a *trip*. I had been very naive going into this, thinking I'd make my way toward some sort of enlightenment. Instead, what I was getting was a full-blown acid trip gone wrong. The sounds of the waves crashing against the shore were so loud by now that I felt a tangible pain pierce my brain. Covering my ears with my hands seemed to make it worse, and the heat of the oil emanating from my wrists made my skin actually sizzle, as if it were on fire. No, I could actually smell it. My skin was burning. I started to panic. *I'm not going to make it through this*, I thought. The realization brought with it a complete sense of terror. The trip was supposed to last all night long, all the way until sunrise, and we had just started. *This is just the beginning. There is no way I'll make it through.* The fear I felt welling up inside of me in that moment was worse than anything I'd ever experienced in my life. It was the feeling of absolute, gut-wrenching regret and a fear so intense I wanted to crawl out of my own skin. I had no idea what I'd gotten myself into, but I knew I was heading somewhere really, really bad. I remembered what Kim had said and threw myself on the floor and into Child's Pose.

The cool tile felt good against my burning hands. I tried to pray. I tried to remember all the good in the world, but I was too exposed, too vulnerable. The sounds surrounding me now were like something out of a horror movie. Lying in Child's Pose, I heard something over by my side. It sounded like critters making their way toward me. I tried to turn my head to look, and in that instant I realized—I was frozen. I tried to move my hands. I couldn't. I tried to get off the floor but my body wasn't cooperating. I was paralyzed. What was it Rodrigo had said? "Te paraliza"—*It will paralyze you.* I screamed for him. He had promised he'd be there. "Rodrigo!" I cried. "Help me! . . . Rodrigo! I can't move! . . . *Rodrigooooooo!!!!!!!!*" Nothing. No one came. It was as if I were all alone in the whole world. I was on my own. Why had I left the safety of my hammock? At least there I was cocooned, safe, but now here I was on the stone floor, exposed to all the dangers of the world. I had made a huge mistake. All of this had been a huge mistake.

In the midst of the horror I heard what sounded like a million cockroaches scattering across the floor. I hate cockroaches and now armies of them were descending on me, crawling over my body and in my hair. I was so immersed in the terror of the situation that I could no longer think about it or objectively assess it—it was 100 percent happening. It was as real as the tile floor beneath me and there was no way to escape. The cockroaches were everywhere. Some made their way into my ears and gnawed into my skull. I could hear them, feel them, smell them. Some crawled up my nose. I was choking on them. I got the urge to vomit as I felt their prickly little legs scatter up and down my throat, but I was chained to the floor. I couldn't move. The next thing I knew I saw dead bodies closing in on me. They were zombie-like, with bones poking through their skin and pieces of flesh hanging from their faces. I could smell the stench of their decay. I sensed that they were desperate to be saved.

The horrors kept coming: spiders with hairy legs and sharp teeth, alien animals, sticky, green vines poking through the floor and wrapping around my ankles to pull me under the soil. All around me was a thick, black mist that made it hard for me to breathe. Worst of all was the all-consuming panic of knowing that I wasn't going to make it out alive. A snake raised up, revealing razor-sharp teeth. *This is the moment I'm going to die*, I thought. I cried for Rodrigo again. "*Rodrigo!!! Ayúdame!*" I had been on the floor for many hours now, enduring the most terrifying, abhorring things. Things I could never have imagined. It was all real. There was no part of me doubting that. It was happening, right here, right now. Suddenly, in the midst of it, out of nowhere, I heard Rodrigo's voice. "Do you need my help?" he asked. "Yes, of course I need your help!" I replied, panicked. "Can't you see I'm dying? I need to get off the floor!" Since I couldn't move, Rodrigo picked me up. He carried me to a sofa in a corner of the room. For a split second I thought the nightmare was over and that I was going to live, but the visions came back with a vengeance: the cockroaches, the decayed bodies, the spiders, the vines, the black mist, the snake—everything at once. All my worst nightmares wrapped up into one hellish experience, enveloped in the knowing that my death was imminent. Getting off the floor had been my one longing, my way out, but now that I was off it I realized it didn't help. There was no way out. I was too exhausted to scream and became overwhelmed with a feeling of hopelessness. I just couldn't fight anymore. *If I'm going to die, I might as well stop fighting*, I thought. I felt death around the corner; it was so close. I knew I wasn't going to make it out alive. *I give up*, I thought. *I surrender. I let go.* And so . . . I did.

Instead of fighting the terrors happening to me, I invited them. I stopped resisting and instead allowed everything to come my way—if there was ever the embodiment of "letting go," this was it. I started welcoming all the horrors. And here is the thing: the moment I let go, the moment I gave in to death, everything changed. It was literally as if I'd flipped a switch—everything went from darkness to sudden bright, shining light. The cockroaches all turned into a flock of white doves and flew away. The vines sprouted into beautiful, long-stemmed daisies. The decaying bodies healed into my loved ones: my sister, my best friend, my grandmother. The snake morphed into my puppy, Quila, wagging her tail. The thick, suffocating mist that had enshrouded me was now a warm, white light and I was glowing from the inside out. Bathed in the light, I felt as if I were in the presence of God. No, I was not just in the presence of God. I was God. There was no difference between us anymore, no separation. I was in the midst of the most intense spiritual awakening of my entire life. All those years I had spent resisting the dark had kept me from the light. The pain isn't the problem, the problems aren't the problem. The resistance is. I felt myself exhale away years, eons, lifetimes of suffering. Everything I'd ever been through had brought me here. All that was left was love. I stayed there, bathing in light, for what felt like an infinite time. It is very hard to put into words the experience I had of surrendering. I've read about it in spiritual texts, but I had never fully understood what it meant to be free. I was whole. At peace. One with God.

When I finally opened my eyes it felt like years had passed. I had become a mother and a grandmother and so many lives had passed, but yet, I was just born. The concept of time seemed very strange. The sun was rising and the sky looked like it was painted in wide brushstrokes of pink, orange, a golden yellow. *Someone created that*, I thought. But it was more than a thought, it was an understanding. At the same instant I realized: I created that. There was no separation between God and me, or between God and any of us. I was alone, but I'd never been more together in my life. I got up and walked barefoot out onto the grass. I looked down and saw the most beautiful shapes moving below me. *What are these magical things?* I thought. It took a while for it to register. My feet! My feet were tan and a little dirty, with tiny blond hairs sprouting from the tops of my toes. I'd never seen something so precious, so beautiful. How were these my feet? I wondered. Have I had these feet all along? I was filled with unconditional love for each of my ten toes. I lifted my head up and gazed at the sky. The beauty I witnessed was unlike anything I'd ever experienced before. My feet. The sky. Everything in between. All of life is so unbelievably precious. How had I not known this all along?

A ravenous hunger overtook me and I headed for the main house, still enthralled and in awe by everything around me. I heard a bark in the distance. Quila! My precious puppy came running. She jumped into my arms and licked my face. The love emanating from her little body was palpable. *How had I not noticed all of this before?* I wondered. Had I been so weighed down by darkness and pain that I didn't recognize the beauty and love surrounding me?

When I entered the house, I found the others gathered around a big table in the garden, enjoying a feast. "There she is!" someone said. John stood and hugged me. "You saved me last night," he said, tears running down his cheeks. "Me too," someone said. "And me!" added a third person. I looked around the table. They were all so beautiful. "What do you mean?" I asked. John tried to explain: The previous night had been gut-wrenching, he said. Everyone was experiencing death and darkness. "I was sure I was going to die," he said. Everyone was. Out of all the experiences the group had had with the medicine, this was the worst by far. Then something happened: A huge bright light emanated from the corner of the room and washed over everyone. "We were all overcome with feelings of peace and calm," John said. "We have been talking about it all morning. We could all pinpoint it from the same place. It was so clear where the light was coming from—it was godlike. It saved us all; it transformed the entire night. When the ceremony was over, the first thing I did was walk over to where the light was coming from. And there you were, on a couch, sleeping." I nodded, understanding fully. I didn't feel any attachment to the idea of my having emanated that light, because I knew it wasn't true. It was our light. Actually, the idea of "me" felt very strange. My perception of the world was morphing—or was I returning to something I had known all along but just forgotten?

Rodrigo explained. "Sometimes one person in the group has a shift big enough to spread to the entire ceremony—like rings on water. That is what happened last night." Rodrigo took a seat next to me. He was so beautiful. Everything made such perfect sense. I hugged him, and felt curiosity bubbling inside me. "Can I ask you something?" I asked in Spanish. "Last night I yelled for you and you didn't come. I spent hours on the floor before you finally came; was that on purpose? Did it have to be that way for the transformation to come?"

Rodrigo looked bewildered. "What do you mean?" he asked. "You called for me and I came right away." Now it was my turn to be confused. "You drank the medicine. I guided you to your hammock, but I stayed close. I knew it was your first time; you are the youngest of the group. Almost right away you got out of your hammock and lay down on the floor. Only a few minutes passed. You called my name and I brought you over to the sofa. You were on the sofa the entire night. Was that not your experience?"

I started smiling, and then a laugh came bubbling up from deep within my belly. Once I started laughing I couldn't stop. I couldn't contain my joy. Before I knew it, we were all laughing, not entirely sure of why but also not needing a reason. When our laughter subsided, my face was aching from smiling so big. The awful visions I'd witnessed the night before, the horror that seemed like a lifetime, had really only been minutes. Rodrigo looked at me with an expression of understanding.

"Que belleza. The night was dark. Then the light came through you," Rodrigo said.

The light I'd discovered during the ceremony stayed with me as we made our way back home. It's stayed with me ever since. I had been shown the lesson of a lifetime. What we resist persists. Whether it's pain, anxiety, fear, loss—whatever emotion you feel—don't fight it. Experience it. Feel it all. Lean into it. Surrender to it. Breathe into it fully. Open your arms wide and welcome it all. *Let go.* It will lead you to the light.

6

RECEIVE

After being in Costa Rica for a year or so I finally got my own house. A proper house! Alright, it was more like a shack. The roof leaked, I didn't have a fridge, a family of scorpions lived in the shower, and when the street flooded, muddy water poured through the front door. I didn't have hot water, electricity was sporadic, and the whole place smelled of dirt and mold. Even so, I was happy there. I woke up every morning before sunrise to the sound of waves crashing on the shore; that's how close I was to the ocean. My days always began with meditation; I'd walk down the beach to one of the deserted lifeguard towers there. Climbing up the steps always filled me with an almost electrical sensation—those mornings were sacred and the life I had created for myself was so simple yet so beautiful that I almost couldn't believe it was mine. I'd settle there, looking out at the ocean as the sun rose, and then close my eyes and sit in meditation for at least an hour. Meditating came as easy as breathing. All I had to do was close my eyes and anchor into my breath, and I'd find myself floating beyond time and space. Quila was always by my side. Sometimes after meditating I'd catch a few waves, or I'd go straight to the fruit stand for breakfast. I practiced yoga every day, too, but yoga asana, the poses, was secondary to meditation for me. Quieting my mind was my priority; moving my body came second. Throughout the day I'd have plenty of good conversation with the backpackers passing through town and found myself immersed in deep conversation everywhere I went. At the time I didn't have a phone, or a computer, or a "real" job. I worked for John and his team, but they would travel for long stretches at a time and then I wouldn't have much to do. I bartended here and there, and waitressed a few days a week, but that barely covered the rent. I was so poor that on some days I had to choose who would eat breakfast: Quila or me. The dog always won. I didn't have much in the way of things, but I had friends and peace of mind, and sun-kissed skin and braids in my hair.

One afternoon, I walked into the dive shop where my friend Laura worked, looking for a hammock and someone to talk to.

"Some hippie girl is trying to steal your boyfriend!" she said before bothering to say hello.

"What boyfriend?" I asked.

"Diego!" she said.

Diego was a Brazilian guy I'd been seeing. A calm, sweet twentysomething neighbor of mine who was living in Costa Rica for the same reason as every other dude with a surfboard— to look for the next perfect wave.

"A girl with brown boots and long hair walked into the shop asking for him," Laura said. "She said they had been dating for a while. She looked kind of like you, except she was shorter, with darker hair, and she didn't wear as many bracelets. A Tica version of you. She seemed nice, but she is dating your boyfriend! Aren't you upset?"

"He's not my boyfriend," I said. I'd been dating Diego casually for a few months, the way I'd casually dated a few other guys since I settled in town. Laura looked at me skeptically. "Sure he's not," she said. "Fine!" I said. "I'll ask him about her."

When I questioned Diego, he said he didn't know what I was talking about and that he wasn't seeing anybody else. I decided the girl was either making up a story or someone I needed to watch out for. Turns out, I didn't have to wait long to find out.

A short time later, I was walking down Sesame Street, the small dirt road lined with houses occupied mostly by expats and long-term visitors, on my way to the beach, when I saw her. I was barefoot, with my puppy on my heels. The girl walking toward me was wearing a cropped top over a flowy purple skirt, and a magnificent pair of boots. Somehow I knew right away that this was the girl Laura had been talking about. Gearing up for confrontation, I was taken aback when she looked at me and smiled.

"Hey! Isn't this the *nicest* day?" she asked, her brown eyes twinkling.

"Hi . . . um . . . yes . . . it is," I said.

"I'm Andrea. Nice to meet you! You're Rachel, right?"

"I am," I said.

We were quiet for a minute and I studied her face. She was incredibly beautiful. If this was the girl who was competing for Diego's affection, I should have been threatened, but for some reason I wasn't.

"I love your dress," Andrea said.

"I like your boots," I replied.

"You can borrow them if you like. Are you going to the beach?" I nodded. "Want some company? I'm really good company. And I have snacks."

It took about five minutes for us to figure out that it was indeed true: we were seeing the same guy. It took even less time for both of us to decide to dump him. We also realized we were neighbors. Andrea had just moved into the house directly next to mine. She planned to stay for what she described as "an infinite amount of mind-blowing time."

Andrea spoke English like an American but laced with Colombian intonation and lots of Costa Rican slang. She said she was born in Colombia and grew up in Costa Rica but went to school in the States, and now she was exploring the country, trying to avoid going to university for as long as she could. She had long, messy chestnut hair, thick, dark eyelashes, and pale skin. She was thin, with curves in all the right places—she was a knockout—but she wasn't preoccupied with her appearance. Her confidence made me think a lot about my perceptions of myself. I am tall, with broad shoulders and long legs, but, unlike Andrea, I was always insecure about my appearance. I never forgot the time that—when I was thirteen and on my way home from school—a construction worker whistled after me and cautioned: "Looking good! Just make sure you don't get anymore meat on those bones!" I was confounded. How much meat was "too much" to have on your bones? When I got home, I went straight to my mom's scale and began a habit of writing down my weight every day to make sure I wasn't gaining. For most of my life, I had always been looking at myself from the outside, picking things apart. It seemed like Andrea had never had an insecure day in her life. If there was a body of water nearby, she was comfortable enough in her skin to throw off all of her clothes to swim butt-naked. After that first day we quickly became inseparable.

She nicknamed me "Macha," which, loosely translated, means "blond" or "Blondie." One day, laying under one of the almond trees by the beach, I found myself thinking, *So this is what real friendship is like?* We'd spent the morning reading in the shade, barely speaking, pausing only to reach for another slice of pineapple or to read something out loud. We didn't have to talk all the time; I didn't have to fill the silence with platitudes or politeness. We could just . . . Be. It was strange, but from the day we met it felt as if we'd known each other for a long, long time. We finished each other's sentences, wore each other's clothes, shared jewelry, braided each other's hair, and gravitated toward the same food, books, songs, and guys. I never had a friend who was so much like a sister; it felt like we were made from the same flesh and blood. Diego became so uncomfortable with our friendship that he ended up leaving town.

After a while, Andrea moved in with me. We were spending all of our waking time together anyway; it didn't make sense to pay for two houses. Within a few months we had a routine: meditating in the mornings, spending time on the beach, going to yoga, cooking, drinking wine, and messing around with the beach guys. She showed me how to build my first altar and how to work with angel cards. She introduced me to palo santo, and ecstatic dance, and the art of making crochet bracelets. She taught me how to follow the rivers to the best waterfalls and how to sing the old grandmother songs. Just like me, Andrea devoured spiritual books and was on a quest for meaning. I'd had many girlfriends in my life, but for some reason, this was the first time that I'd ever felt truly safe in a relationship, which brought a lot of realizations about my previous friendships. I knew it wasn't about my old friends—it was about the old me. I always had a hard time letting people in—I didn't trust easily—and often kept people away or created drama. I was reliving many of my challenging relationship patterns with my mother in my female relationships, always waiting for the other person to leave me. It wasn't until I met Andrea that I realized what sisterhood could actually be. Our time together was sacred—my soul grew with her. The love I felt for her and the ease of our friendship was different from any relationship I'd ever experienced. Before Andrea, I never had a friend I felt I could completely trust. I often created problems in my friendships in order to give myself a reason to leave before someone left me. I didn't know that friendship required intimacy and vulnerability, from both sides. Andrea wasn't afraid to show affection or open herself up. She loved to cuddle—she was very touchy-feely and would always hold my hand or my arm or play with my hair. With time, those qualities I admired so much began to rub off on me. The more we got to know each other, the more we realized we had in common. For the year that followed, everyone in town knew that wherever I went, Andrea was close by, and wherever Andrea went, I was sure to be by her side. When some tourists at a bar told us, "Gosh, you look so much alike! Are you twins?" we started calling each other *gemela*, for twin. Actually, we looked nothing alike. I was tall and blond and she was short and brunette. But there was something there that was so similar, we got used to people asking us if we were sisters. In a way, we were. It was like we'd always been.

I dated along the way: Luigi, a local guy from San José whose heart I ended up breaking but who later became one of my closest guy friends. And Brock, who'd come to Costa Rica from Portland, Oregon, in search of the perfect wave. I loved each of them but I was physically and emotionally incapable of committing and always moved on to someone else. My fear of commitment extended to every part of my life. For instance, I never fully gave up my apartment in Sweden. Two years into my stay in Costa Rica I had managed to save up enough money for a trip back to Europe. I boarded a plane and slipped back into my life in Uppsala for a few weeks while Andrea watched over Quila and our little place on the beach.

While it was great to see family and old friends again, I couldn't wait to get back to Dominical. Sweden hadn't felt like home in a long time. After a Christmas celebration, my father invited me to join him and my little sister on a vacation to Aruba. It was on my way back to Costa Rica so I willingly said yes. I'd never even heard of Aruba before but I loved the island right away. It had the tropical vibe of Costa Rica, the gorgeous beaches, the warm water, the sunshine, and the laid-back lifestyle, but it was ordered and structured in a way that reminded me of Sweden. The roads were solid (unlike in Costa Rica, where the roads washed away every rainy season), the water was safe to drink, health care was good, and crime was virtually nonexistent.

I spent the first two days in Aruba with my dad and sister lounging on the beach and playing in the sea. Andrea sent me a text. You're just a short plane ride away now! She missed me. Looking out at the most turquoise sea I'd ever seen, I suddenly felt no rush to head back to Costa Rica. Aruba was gorgeous. Who knows, maybe I'll meet a cute Caribbean guy and stay a little longer! I wrote back. I was joking—I was already in the middle of a challenging breakup and she knew all about it. Funny, she answered. Stop breaking hearts and hurry back home. She was right. I needed to be alone.

One morning Dad and I decided to pop into a surf shop in town. I walked in and literally straight into a tall, blond, crazy-handsome guy.

"Hey," he said, towering over me.

My face burned red and I could barely get words out. It took a long moment for me to realize he was reaching his hand out to greet me. I finally took it. "I'm Dennis. Are you okay?" I nodded. "Rachel," I said. I don't know what was happening to me, but I just couldn't get the words to come out. *Who was this guy?* Dennis ended up talking to my dad, who at one point turned to me and asked, "Weren't you looking for a surf instructor, Rachel?" To which Dennis responded by scribbling his number down on a piece of paper and hand-ing it to me. "Call me if you want to go surfing. I'd love to take you."

"Th-thanks," I said, mortified.

Where was my normal, breezy self? I wondered. I couldn't string two words together! I couldn't wait to get away. Dennis smiled at me as I walked out, but I couldn't even look at him. I was stricken. Dad was exasperated. "You have the *worst* taste in men," he said once we got outside. "Just look at that guy in there! Humble, straightforward, good-looking. You could tell right away, that's a great guy. And you didn't even give him the time of day!"

If only he knew.

A week passed and every day I'd wake up thinking about the guy in the surf shop. I couldn't pinpoint what it was, but I couldn't get him out of my head. Just the thought of seeing him again was ridiculous—I was on a tiny island in the middle of nowhere that I'd never set foot on again! I focused my atten-tion on my family and the beautiful ocean, but every morning I woke up thinking of him. When Dad left to take a short jaunt to Colombia, I finally mustered up the courage to go back to the store. *What's the harm?* I thought. *I'm just going to go say hi. No big deal.* With my little sister, Emelie, in tow, I hailed a taxi and we headed for downtown. I felt like I was on the cusp of doing something big, and it terrified me. So I made a wager with the universe. *If there is any reason why this is not meant to be, give me a sign and I'll trust it.*

We arrived downtown and found that everything was

closed. Apparently, Aruba shuts down on Sundays. Dejected, we took the taxi back to our hotel, but I couldn't get that guy out of my head.

That wasn't a sign, I told myself. *Everything just happened to be closed! I'll try again tomorrow.* The next day I convinced my sister to go with me again. And I wagered with the universe—again. *If for some reason this isn't meant to be, give me another sign and this time I'll take it seriously.* We got to the store and . . . Dennis wasn't there. My heart sank. His coworkers were all present, however.

"You never called Dennis!" one exclaimed. "He really thought you would call!"

I thought I would die from embarrassment. They had clearly been talking about me during the week, and there I was, back in the shop with my nine-year-old sister, trying to act casual while five surf dudes stared at me.

"He's in the office upstairs," one said. *This is not a sign*, I thought to myself. *Not a sign.* "Oh, that's fine, we're just shopping a little!" I said.

I lingered for as long as I could, looking at things I wasn't at all interested in, pretending to need all sorts of stuff I didn't need. Finally, after what felt like forever, Dennis appeared.

"You came back," he said.

"Yes," I said. "I needed . . . board shorts."

"You so do not!" Emelie cried. "You already have board shorts! Like, a ton of them!"

I shot her a look that I hoped said, "If you don't shut the hell up, you're not getting ice cream *ever again*."

"Alright, well, I'm here if you need me," Dennis said, stepping behind the counter.

That's it? I wondered. *He's not going to talk to me? Or ask me out? Why was the universe making me work so hard to see this guy?* I felt too embarrassed to ask him out in front of all of his friends, so I ended up paying for our things and we left.

As I was walking across the open-air mall, I felt someone looking at me. I turned and saw Dennis, hanging on to the doorframe of the shop and leaning out, watching me walk away. I mustered the courage to flash him a huge smile (a pretty obvious one!) and kept walking. I'd promised my sister we'd get something to eat, so we sat down at a restaurant. Dennis suddenly appeared. Now he was the one who looked nervous.

"Hey! I don't know if you're busy . . . maybe you are . . . but I'm off in twenty minutes and I was going to go check out the waves. Want to come?" he asked.

"Surf? Me? Yes! Sure! Definitely!" I said, a little too excitedly.

"Unless you're just sitting down to eat?" he said.

"Eat? Us? No, noooo . . . not at all. We're not eating! Let's go surf," I said.

"What do you mean we're not eating?" my sister cried, waving her menu at me. "You said we were going to eat here! I'm starving!"

Oh God. Emelie. Just. Be. Quiet. "I'll take you to the hotel," I said in Swedish. "Dad will be back by now. I'll get you ice cream and you can watch a movie in the room. Please just be cool!"

"Oh . . . you like this guy! Now I get it!" she said in Swedish. "Okay, fine. But don't forget about my ice cream."

We dropped Emelie off with Dad, and Dennis and I drove to the beach. The surf was too big for me and the break was crowded with local surfers fighting for the best waves.

"Are you okay to chill here?" Dennis asked.

"Yes, sure," I said.

With that, my new acquaintance jumped out of the car and started taking off his clothes. Like, all of his clothes. We'd only just met and here he was, stark naked, changing right in front of me? *What is he doing?* I wondered. I'd never known someone so comfortable in his own skin, and for a moment I thought about Andrea and her ability to get naked at the drop of a dime. *They would really get along,* I thought. A vision of the three of us walking down a beach flashed in front of my eyes. I shook it off—where was my mind going? I'd known this guy for five minutes! A second later Dennis was in his board shorts and headed for the water.

I sat on the shore and watched him until the sun set. As he paddled back in, I felt butterflies in my stomach. Why was I feeling so nervous? It wasn't like he was the first cute surfer guy I'd ever hung out with. He was just one guy in a string of many whom I'd flirted with that year—it had definitely been the most exciting year of my life in the boy department. Most of them had been surfers, just like him. Why was I feeling so . . . awkward?

Dennis dried himself off and sat down next to me on the beach.

"Want to go for something to eat?" he asked.

We ended up at a Thai place and sat for hours, eating vegetable rolls and yellow curry, drinking Singhas, and talking. Neither of us wanted the night to end.

When finally the restaurant started closing up, we reluctantly got up to pay the bill. We stood outside the restaurant, neither of us wanting to leave. "Want to go for a drive?" he asked. Silly question. We drove with the windows down, his hand on the clutch, my feet on the dashboard. We got to a lookout and stepped out of the car. What looked like a thousand lights glittered in the distance. Suddenly we were out of words. He stepped closer and for the longest time we stood like that, close, but not touching. I felt like I was on the cusp of something momentous. Part of me knew: *If I kiss this man there's no turning back.*

"Maybe we'll see some shooting stars," Dennis said as we stood and looked up at the sparkling canvas. "I've never seen one," I said.

It was true. In all my nights spent traveling, I'd never once caught a shooting star. Andrea used to call me bad luck. "We never see them when Macha is around!" she'd say whenever we gathered on the beach for bonfires at night. Well. Standing there on that lookout, on a small Caribbean island that I'd probably never set foot on ever again, I decided to make one final wager with the universe. *If we see a shooting star, I'll kiss him.* A second later a star shot across the sky, leaving a long trail of bright orange glitter behind. In an instant, our lips met. I don't know who kissed whom, but he tasted like salt water and sunshine.

After five beautiful days together, it was time for me to

return to Costa Rica. By then I had been gone for a while and Andrea had taken Quila from the beach in Dominical to San José. I was embarrassed. I'd literally just taken off on a whim and left my whole life behind. I felt so irresponsible. Andrea didn't seem to mind. She was stoked to see me.

We decided to spend a week back in Dominical. I'd assumed that while I was there, I'd try to get a new house to rent and start working at the bar again.

Our time at the beach was epic. I was back in my element, with the person I loved most in the world. We meditated every morning, went to the waterfalls, swam naked, sang, chanted, and played with the dogs—Andrea's two and my Quila. Our evenings were spent hanging out with our old friends, dancing, sitting around fires. Life was good.

Still, every day I thought about Dennis, but I couldn't imagine what we had working out. We hadn't spoken since I'd left Aruba two weeks earlier—who knew if he was even thinking about me? One morning I woke up from a dream about him—again—and told Andrea about it.

"Call him!!!" she said. "See what happens. Part of me feels like you just need to chill and be alone. But this guy! What is it about this guy? You are dreaming about him every night. Just call him. Let the universe decide what's next."

I didn't have a phone, so I took a few hundred colones and walked to a pay phone across the street. I dialed Dennis's number. My hands turned sweaty when the phone started ringing. He picked up right away. Just hearing his voice made my heart race.

"Hey, it's Rachel!" I said. "I've been thinking about you."

"I've been thinking about you, too," he said. "A lot."

My face flushed. He *had* been thinking about me!

"So, I was thinking, maybe I'll come back to see you?" I said, holding my breath.

"Yeah, that would be good," he replied.

"Tomorrow?" I asked, half joking.

"Yes, tomorrow is good! I'll pick you up at the airport?"

"See you soon," I said, hanging up.

From where I stood, I could see Andrea waiting on our balcony.

"I'm going to Aruba!" I shouted.

She ran down the stairs and jumped me in the street. "*Aruba! Aruba! Aruba!*" we shouted, bouncing up and down.

I booked a flight for the next morning, before I got the chance to change my mind. Andrea and I drove back from the beach to San José that same night, arriving very late. We shared her bed and I woke up in the morning with her arm in my face. When she dropped me off at the airport I got strangely emotional. I was on my way to Aruba to be with some guy I barely knew, when I could have stayed there and continued my life with her, my best friend.

Andrea grabbed my shoulders and looked me in the eyes. "This is all going to be amazing," she said. "Trust it."

I relaxed, but only a little. "But what if he's some kind of psychopath?" I asked.

"Well. If he is a psychopath, he's a really cute one."

Leave it to Andrea. We hugged, and I was off.

7
___

LISTEN

Dennis was waiting for me at arrivals, wearing a bright green T-shirt. We hugged and headed to his place, a little house he rented with his best friend, Cado. Things between us got intense quickly, but it was an entirely different feeling from the infatuations I'd experienced before. For the first time, I didn't feel the need to run, or go looking for the next thing. Lying in Dennis's arms at night, I could feel my body relax in a way it never had. I felt at home. At peace. Dennis felt like an anchor in my messy life.

I'd only been living on the island for about a month when I saw a tiny puppy in a trash can on the side of the road. I figured him to be two or three weeks old. His legs looked like tooth-picks, his belly was swollen, and his fur was dirty and matted. I fell instantly in love. I brought the puppy home, fed and bathed him, and left him in an open moving box with a note for Dennis: "Don't get angry—we'll discuss it later."

I didn't know how he would react—we'd only been dating for a month—but when I got back home I found Dennis sitting with the puppy on his lap, tears in his eyes. It had been love at first sight for him, too. We tried to decide on a name for our new little family member. Dennis wanted to name him Dynamite; I liked Yogi. We settled on Sgt. Pepper (Pepper for short) after our favorite Beatles album. Dennis's dog, Laika, loved the puppy, too. Poor Cado. Living with two dogs and a couple who were newly in love was not what he had bargained for and soon he found a place of his own.

While I figured out what I wanted to do with my life, I took two part-time jobs, as a server and a bartender. After a few weeks of my working nights while Dennis worked days, we decided it wasn't working—we barely saw each other. I went to the beach to meditate on what I really wanted to do or "be." *What did I truly love?* I asked myself. If I was going to settle on this island and spend several hours a day working, it had to be something that brought me joy. The answer that came to me was undeniable. Yoga. I wanted to teach yoga. My yoga practice had become a huge part of my life and every morning I would roll my mat out on our little patio to stretch and move with my breath. I'd already taught some classes in Costa Rica and could feel a dream forming. What if I could teach yoga for a living?

I got a job working in reception at a small studio on the island and slowly began teaching some classes, using books and senior teachers to guide me. Eventually I got a job teaching at a resort, and with time, my classes got so popular I was promoted to yoga director of the hotel. I completely immersed myself in the yoga world. I didn't have any official training, but the sum of my book learning, personal practice, classes, and workshops had paid off. Teaching came easy to me; it felt like something I was supposed to have been doing all along. The next step was training to get certified.

By then, I had been in Aruba for nine whole months. The course I chose was in Costa Rica. With the blessing of my employer, I signed up to go and flew on the return ticket I'd never used when I left Costa Rica to see Dennis, thinking I would soon return. My plan was to stay with Andrea before my three-week teacher training in the jungle, after which Dennis would meet me for vacation, and then we had planned to pack up my things and return to Aruba with Quila.

I got to San José and Andrea picked me up at the airport. I was so happy to see her. We spoke on Skype all the time and texted almost every day, but I'd missed spending quality time with my best friend. We spent the next few days together, hashing out the details of her latest relationship and mine with Dennis. "Remember when you worried that maybe he was a psychopath?" she reminded me. We both laughed. I thought about how quickly my life had shifted. And something within me had shifted, too; something Andrea noticed. I was calmer, steadier, she said. Having Dennis in my life had helped to ground me.

When it was time for me to leave for my training, Andrea dropped me off at the bus station and I set off to my next adventure. I was super excited, and nervous to start teacher training. It took place at a retreat center in Puerto Viejo, on the Caribbean side of the country. I walked to the first session, giddy with anticipation. The deck was in the middle of the jungle and we were a group of thirty women, sitting mat to mat in a circle. When the teacher walked in, the atmosphere felt almost holy.

Lori was in her fifties, with hair that was pulled back in a tight knot. She greeted us, then sat on her mat and placed her hands together at her heart in anjali mudra, the heart before the heart. The room was silent. Right as she was about to speak, she noticed a bug on her mat and smashed it. *Whack!* I gasped. The teacher killed a bug!? On her yoga mat? I'd always felt an innate reverence for animals and insects and never even killed a mosquito. The first of the five yamas, the moral, ethical, and societal guidelines for yogis, is ahimsa—the practice of non-harm. Surely that included bugs! I knew right then that I had the wrong teacher. It was downhill from there.

I always advise people who are looking for a new teacher to find one with whom they can imagine meeting for a cup of tea. For me, that was not Lori. One day she was talking about the challenges of being a yoga instructor and used me as an example. "Some of you are going to have to learn some hard lessons," she said. "Rachel, for instance, is going to have to learn that there is more to yoga than just looking pretty." All eyes turned to me. My face was burning. *Yoga was more than looking pretty? What? Why did she think that of me?* I owned all of two pairs of yoga pants, never wore any makeup, and kept my long hair tied back for practice. I didn't understand why she would talk about me in that way, but I was deeply wounded by her comment and spent the rest of the training trying to divert attention from myself while sticking to the program.

Every day of the two-hundred-hour course had a theme so we could immerse ourselves in different styles of yoga. I was most curious about Kundalini. I remembered what Kim, the Kundalini teacher from the farm who'd attended the ayahuasca ceremony with me, said about it. The practice consisted of a repetition of simple poses and intense breath work that released powerful energy from the spine up through the crown of the head, merging with the divine and, if we're lucky, resulting in enlightenment. "It can be overwhelming, and there are too many people teaching who shouldn't be," Kim had said.

I'd learned that Lori taught Kundalini infrequently and I was nervous when we stepped on our mats. The group dynamic was off—I didn't feel safe. We started moving, doing simple poses in repetition. I immersed myself in my body and breath and before I knew it, I'd lost track of time. At the end of the practice we were seated in meditation, and I felt as if my hands and feet were on fire—similar to the feeling I'd had during the cacao ceremony. An intense sadness came over me and I started having visions. Suddenly I saw people I'd lost throughout my life descending from above, landing on the yoga deck in front of me: my stepfather, Stefan, who died in the plane crash; my grandfather on my mother's side, who'd passed away before I was born; Marianne, my mom's stepmother, who'd lost her battle with cancer when I was a teenager. When I tried to reach for them, they moved farther away. Overcome with deep feelings of grief and despair, I began to cry so hard I couldn't breathe. I lost connection with the earth below me and felt myself being swallowed up by a dark, gray cloud.

When I opened my eyes again, three hours had passed. It was almost dark and the deck was empty. I gathered my things and walked toward the retreat center. I was almost back when I heard a voice call to me.

"Hey! You!"

I lifted my gaze and saw a woman standing on the steps of a neighboring cabin. I recognized her as the resident healer. She worked at the center giving massages and doing energy work.

"Do you want to come in for a second?" she asked.

I nodded, almost in a daze, and slowly walked up the steps. She ushered me inside and to the back of the cabin.

"Lie down," she said, pointing to a soft table.

I laid on my back and she started chanting and working on me with crystals and essential oils. Little by little, I started feeling normal again. When it was over, she invited me to stay for tea.

"What happened to you?" she asked. "I saw you walk by . . . I *felt* you walk by. I've never felt such low, heavy energy surrounding a person. I'm not sure what happened to you, but you were not in your body at all. And not in a good way."

I explained about the Kundalini session: the visions I'd had and the feeling of despair that overcame me. She was angry.

"That is so irresponsible!" she cried. "These are sensitive energies to mess with. And they just left you like that? No one to support you? All alone?"

"Yes," I said.

The woman looked deeply troubled. "Some people are very sensitive to this type of work and can easily drop into the Kundalini energy," she said. "It's clear that you are such a person. With time and practice you'll learn how to harness it and turn it toward light, but for someone who is inexperienced, you can become overwhelmed and swallowed up by it."

I listened intently as she continued. "It seems to me that you have a very strong ability to connect with the other side—a good quality to have, but without direction, it can be outright dangerous. Promise me: Never move into this type of work without making sure you resonate with your teacher."

"I promise," I said.

I finished the teacher training a few days later with my certificate in hand, having learned a critical lesson. Trust what your body tells you when you encounter a new person. If your gut reaction tells you it isn't right, follow that instinct. And most important: do your research before investing in anything that relates to your heart. Listening to your intuition takes practice and sometimes we have to move into a gray area to truly figure out where our boundaries are. I will never study under a teacher I don't trust deeply ever again, but I'm grateful for the lessons it brought me.

Dennis met up with me in San José and finally got to meet Andrea for the first time when we picked him up at the airport. It was a big moment—my best friend meeting the man of my dreams—and I was anxious. What if they didn't like each other? Dennis kissed me, then picked up Andrea in a big bear hug.

"Finally we meet!" he said.

In the car, we talked and laughed as if it had always been the three of us. In just a few hours, they had developed their own inside jokes—many at my expense.

"What's it like living with a person who chews with her mouth open all the time?" Andrea asked, elbowing Dennis.

He rolled his eyes. "I thought I was the only one who noticed! It drives me *crazy*! She chews like she has nuts and bolts in her mouth! It's so loud!"

I pretended to be offended, but I was thrilled. They were acting like brother and sister.

"He is so handsome," Andrea said when we were alone. "I love him! He is the one for you! Do you feel it?"

"I do," I said, blushing.

She rested her head on my shoulder. "Does this mean you're never coming back?" she asked. "No more gemela time?"

We both wiped away tears.

"You're my best friend," I said. "I'll never be far."

At the end of my stay, Dennis and I gathered up Quila and headed home to Aruba with a renewed sense of purpose: we really were a couple now. I hadn't just showed up to visit and stayed with him—I'd actually made the commitment. I even had my dog. We moved to the cutest little place surrounded by a huge garden with three mango trees, a large patio, and palm trees lining the house. We were a family. Dennis, me, and our dogs.

8

GROUND

Dennis and I spent the next year in total bliss. Yet for all of the good that was happening in my life, bad things seemed to follow me. I hadn't had much contact with my family after I left Sweden, except for occasional phone calls. My sisters, who were young kids when I left, were growing up quickly. Hedda was newly into her teenage years and, according to my mom, not doing well. She was drinking and suffered from bouts of depression. Mom called crying one day to tell me that Hedda had tried to kill herself. I was devastated. "I think she needs to come see you for a while," my mother said. "She needs her big sister now, and some sunshine." I loved my baby sister and said that of course she could come. My history, after all, was one of trying to rescue others, and I felt especially responsible for my siblings.

When Hedda arrived I couldn't believe my eyes. Her skin was so pale it was almost blue, and she had dark circles under her eyes. She wore heavy black makeup and her hair was dyed bright turquoise. I ran up to her in the arrivals hall at the air-

port and squeezed her tight. Choking back tears, I held on to
her tiny body, but she barely hugged me back. I was stunned
when we got into the car and she took off her sweater, revealing angry red scars on her arms. They looked like the lines in a
notebook. Hedda was cutting herself. I looked away, trying to
focus on the road.

"Are you happy to be here?" I asked.

"I don't know," she said.

I didn't know how, but I was determined to make her feel
better.

For the next two weeks, Dennis and I showered Hedda
with attention. We swam in the ocean, ate good food, and cud-
dled with the dogs. I tried to get her to join my yoga classes on
the beach, but she always sat off to the side and just stared out
at the water. For the first week, when I asked her questions, she
gave me vague answers. A breakthrough came at the beginning
of the second week.

"I don't feel good at home," she said one day. "I just feel
sad, all the time."

"I'm here for you," I said. "Do you want to talk about
where it's coming from?"

She sighed and looked away. "No. I just want to be with you."

Our time together passed too quickly, but it seemed to have
done Hedda some good. By the time I took her to the airport
to go home, she was tan and the scars on her arms had faded.
She seemed lighter and happier.

"You're okay, right?" I asked before she boarded the plane.

"Yes," she said, smiling. "I just needed a break from everything. I'm fine."

We said our I-love-yous and hugged good-bye. Watching Hedda walk to the gate, I felt a heaviness in the pit of my stomach.

"She's fine," Dennis said, trying to reassure me. "You saw how happy she was this last week. Everything is okay."

"You're right," I said.

I felt I had done everything I could to make Hedda happy. Still, I couldn't help but wonder if it was enough.

Hedda was only back in Stockholm for a day when she tried to jump off a tall building. It took hours for the police to talk her down. When Mom called to tell me, something inside of me broke. The negative voice in the back of my head that I'd been able to keep at bay for so long came back, and with a vengeance. I had failed my little sister on an epic level. If I were a better sister, she wouldn't have tried to kill herself. It was my fault that she wanted to die.

Hedda started seeing a therapist after that. I, on the other hand, decided it was time to start partying. I stopped meditating and spent a lot of time with new friends I'd met, clubbing and drinking. At first I went out once or twice a week, then I was at the bar every day. Dennis was perplexed. This was a version of me he had never seen before—it was a version of me I thought I'd let go of long ago. I felt like I was sixteen again, avoiding my feelings with bottles of tequila. He tried to keep up but always went home early. To be honest, I didn't want him with me. I wanted to be alone with my new friends. Friends who didn't know me and didn't ask questions.

Dennis eventually stopped asking if I wanted him to come

along. Rather than question me about what was going on, he became quiet and distant.

On the surface, I seemed to be having the time of my life—dancing, drinking, and partying every night. I told myself, *I'm living the best of both worlds—just because I teach yoga doesn't mean I have to be a purist!* Deep down, I knew something was deeply off, but I refused to confront my pain and instead numbed myself with alcohol and other distractions.

As days turned to weeks, Dennis and I drifted further and further apart. Inevitably, I met someone else. He was a pretty average guy, the manager of one of the nightclubs I frequented. His name was Miguel; he was from Mexico but had spent the last couple of years in Aruba. He was a photographer; charismatic, fun, and, most important of all, "spiritual." At least that was my perception. The one thing, if I had to find one, that I felt was missing with Dennis was a sense of spirituality. He was a no-nonsense kind of guy, feet on the ground, humble and down-to-earth, but he would never have called himself spiritual. He wasn't into meditation the way I was, and he didn't talk about things like the meaning of life the way Miguel did.

Over the course of the next two months, I got involved with Miguel. We spoke every day, texted, and met at the bar. I lied to Dennis about where I was and whom I was with. I was confused and sad. The further into the deep end with Miguel I got, the more I alienated Dennis. We stopped communicating and started fighting over little stuff. After weeks of my creating a bigger mess than I knew what to do with, my solution was to leave it all and run away. I told Dennis I needed a break to think things over. I wasn't sure about our relationship anymore.

I went home to Sweden and spent most of the time there crying. I stopped communicating with Miguel and began having long talks with my mom. When I said I was contemplating breaking up with Dennis, she started to cry. "Oh, honey," she said. "Please don't make the same mistakes I did. You don't have to run from love.

"Dennis is the best thing that has ever happened to you," she said. "Maybe," I replied. "I just don't think he gets me. He doesn't meditate; he doesn't contemplate the universe like I do. I don't know if this is right." Mom didn't mince words. "Are you crazy?" she asked, exasperated. "He is the most spiritual guy I've ever known! He doesn't have to meditate—he gets it already. You don't have to walk around contemplating the universe all the time unless you are unsure of it. Dennis isn't unsure. He is here, present. You are just trying to find something wrong with him so you can run away."

I wasn't convinced. I told her about Miguel and our flirtation. She instantly became wary and cautioned me. "I want you to think very carefully about what you do next," my mother said. "This decision is going to affect the rest of your life. This other guy . . . it's an illusion. It's not real. Intuitively, I know it's wrong. Dennis is right for you. You know it. I know it. You're meant to be together."

For the two weeks I was in Sweden, I went back and forth about what to do. I spoke to Dennis once or twice. He was heartbroken. How did we go from being in such a good place to uncertainty and total mistrust? I felt guilty causing him so much pain. At the end of my stay in Sweden, I was no clearer about what I wanted, but a part of me had already settled on leaving him. I didn't deserve him, I told myself. He's too good for me. I should get back on the road, move to a new place, find a new guy. The evening before my flight back, I called. Dennis had changed from being sad and distraught to cold and distant. I heard laughter in the background. "Where are you?" I asked. "Out," he said flatly. "With who?" I asked. "You left me, remember?" he replied bitterly. "Why do you even care?" I felt a tightening in my stomach. "I'm flying back tomorrow," I said. "Back to what?" Dennis asked. "I don't know," I said. The line went quiet. "I'm not going to force you to stay with me," Dennis said. "Do what you want to do." His words stung. "Can you pick me up at the airport?" I asked. He paused before answering. "Fine," he said. The line went dead.

My dad lived close to the airport, so I stayed with him the night before my morning flight. "What happened between you and Dennis?" he asked. "It's just not working anymore," I said. Dad wouldn't let it go. "I don't believe that," he said. "Dennis is an awesome guy. You have been so happy with him. Could it be something in *you* that isn't working anymore?" My father had hit a nerve. My face flushed with anger and I lashed out. "Who are you to give me advice?" I asked. "You have four kids with three women, and all of them hate you!" He looked stunned. I had hurt him deeply. "Maybe I don't want that for you," he said, his voice cracking. "Maybe there is something you can learn from my mistakes. Don't be so quick to walk away from something that's good." Hot tears fell from my eyes. "Stop trying to get involved in my life," I cried. "Just leave me the hell alone." I ran upstairs, crying so hard I could barely breathe. *How did I get here?* I wondered. Again, I felt like a teenager. I was being totally unreasonable and I had nowhere to call home. No one to hold me and tell me everything would be okay. I'd never felt so alone.

At the depth of my despair, my computer pinged with a message. *Dennis?* I wondered. My jaw dropped when my eyes hit the screen. It was a message from Dennis's ex-girlfriend Lauren. We'd never spoken before, but from what I had gathered, she absolutely hated me. Dennis had broken things off with her to be with me and their relationship had ended very badly. Why was she writing me?

Hi Rachel,

I think I've started this e-mail a hundred times in the past few weeks and never had the guts to finish it. All I know is that I have to reach out to you or else I'll give myself a big face slap. I treated you so meanly two years ago, when you met Dennis. I judged you, said awful things about you, and went behind your back and did a terrible thing. I didn't know you and I thought you were ruining my life on purpose. And I want to apologize for all of that. I am so very sorry. After Dennis, I was so angry. I hated my life back home and I didn't know what to do about it. I was looking for someone to save me from the awfulness that was my own life, and I felt like you ruined my chance and that it was all your fault (ohmigod, seriously. So immature of me). About 5 months after he broke up with me, I got tired of waiting for someone to rescue me, took a break from my job, traveled to Asia, and got certified to teach yoga (never intending to teach, only wanting to deepen my practice). And since then, in the past two years, I've really started looking at my life in a way that I never did before. I've started being open, and forgiving, and I'm trying to be more honest with myself. I've really started moving toward what I want. I'm working on creating a lifestyle that I love, in a place that I love, with a person that I love. It gets overwhelming at times, not knowing if this step is the right one, or the next step is the right one, or the one after that. But I know that I have to keep going in order to figure out what it is that I'm meant to do. And, oddly, if you never existed, and never had met Dennis, none of that would have happened. So why am I writing you? Because you inspire me so much. After I got done being mad, and realizing how much I needed to get my own shit together, I started looking at your Facebook page. You moved to Aruba and you're making your own life. You did all of the things I wanted to do two years ago, but never had the balls to. And I want to say thank you. For constantly inspiring people all over the world, including myself, and for just being you. It's so huge how you've grown your practice and the yoga community in Aruba. When I was there it was nonexistent and I remember bitching about it constantly. And there you go, not bitching, but doing something about it. I have been teaching yoga all summer to teenage girls, and have my first audition in an actual studio on Friday, which is why I was thinking about you. I have been feeling really called to teach lately, and I'm so excited (and nervous) to be given the opportunity. I know if it is meant to be, it will. And if it isn't, there's something else out there for me. Anyway, thank you so much for changing my life (for the better! Even though I didn't know it) and, oddly, inspiring me far more than you may realize. I hope that we can be friends one day (is that weird? I think it might be a little weird. I don't care). Your courage, your authenticity, and even your style are deeply inspiring to me. Part of me wishes I would have met you instead of Dennis, but the universe works in mysterious ways, doesn't it?

Lauren

I was stunned. Dennis's ex-girlfriend was quite literally the very last person I ever expected to hear from. As far as I knew, she hated me. But here she was writing to me, telling me her story and sending me love. And she was following my Facebook page? I had started one dedicated to my yoga journey just a few months earlier, sharing my class schedule and posting some photos here and there. I couldn't believe it. Somehow, she'd saved me from myself at exactly the right moment. I snapped out of my misery and wrote her back immediately:

This is so totally nuts. You have no idea. I don't know where to start or what to say or what to do right now other than say thank you. Thank you, thank you, thank you. The reason you didn't write me this email days ago is that I needed this so badly, at this exact moment. Not then. Now. I am in the worst space I have been in years, and tonight was the peak of three of the most difficult months I have ever gone through. It's a fun little mix of family drama, alcoholism, and a pretty serious spiritual crisis. Fun stuff. Oh, and me and Dennis have broken up, or are breaking up, or something along those lines. Things are shit and I couldn't take it so I ran away to Sweden for two weeks. I'm sure you're not in any way interested in hearing about that and I won't bore you with details, but the fact that you are writing me this now is amazing and beautiful and also so sad in a way that makes me want to cry. Tonight is my last night in Sweden and I'm in an even bigger mess now than when I left Aruba. I was literally sitting on my bedroom floor crying feeling completely useless and alone when my phone made a funny noise and it's you. Of all people. Writing me these beautiful words and letting me in on your journey and the fact that somehow I have a part in it too. Reminding me that hard times are here for the best reasons, and we need them. I am so, so glad I have been an inspiration to you. You're brave, and totally the cool chick I imagined you to be. I mean, anything else would be weird; we both fell for the same awesome guy. Actually, you're the only one out of the two of us that didn't steal him away, so I think you score way higher on the cool chick scale than I do. I know things were bad back then, and I didn't know you and what happened wasn't ideal. I'm sorry he hurt you, and reading this I am also so very happy that he did. All of my most important realizations and places of growth have happened thanks to really shitty and traumatic situations. I've been blessed with many of them, and I've learnt to accept and be grateful for the fact that they were there. Even if it hurt. Actually, the more it hurt the more I grew and eventually learned to let go, and I know that everything comes our way because we need it. Or, I used to know. I think I've forgotten this most important realization during these past months, and your email just helped to bring all of it back. If I didn't need this pain it wouldn't be here. I feel in no way inspiring or courageous or authentic right now sitting on a bedroom floor in a country that isn't mine anymore, and I feel very very far away from the person you see in me. She's in there somewhere though. Thank you for reminding me that this, too, shall pass. I'm so glad you're here. Super fucking amazing that you are teaching! Really. If you feel it, it's right, and you'll nail the audition I'm sure. Just be you and your classes will rock. Dennis always said he thinks you and me would make the best friends. And now I think so too. Is it weird if we are? Probably. Yes. I don't care. Thank you, for being so cool. I'm going to get up off this floor now.

Rachel

Something in me changed after that. I realized I had been living in a haze—I wasn't actually living at all. How had I gone from living the best years of my life—with the love of my life— to creating such a giant mess? It was like a lightbulb went off in my head and I could finally connect the dots. After my sister's attempted suicide, something inside of me had shattered. I'd spent the months since manifesting that hurt in everything around me, including the most valuable relationship of my life—with Dennis. Being a "rescuer" was so ingrained in my identity that failing my sister brought out every last piece of insecurity from deep inside of me. I had been self-sabotaging ever since, feeling like I wasn't worthy of anything good. Getting that message from his ex-girlfriend, someone who should have absolutely disliked me, pulled me from the murkiness of my sadness and toward the light. There was a synchronicity to the universe and I'd completely lost sight of it. Her story brought me back. The guy she loved dumped her for me, and that heartbreak had sent her on a path that led to a beautiful life of abundance and love. Of course! I knew how it worked. Our most profound discoveries are sparked in darkness, if only we allow ourselves to see them. Dark times come to shake things up and give us the opportunity to get back on track.

It was suddenly clear to me that my flirtation with Miguel had nothing to do with wanting a relationship with him; not at all. Now I could see him in a realistic light and I was disgusted with myself. What road had I been walking down? I felt a fear grip my throat. I was close to losing Dennis. My reason for wanting to leave him—that he wasn't spiritual enough—was far from legitimate. I had needed a reason to leave, and if not that, I would have made up something else. My role since childhood had been that of savior. I was brought up with the notion that I was here to save my mother and that spread to everyone else. Yet I'd failed with my own sister. As a result of that failure, my self-worth was crushed. Subconsciously I'd decided I wasn't worthy of happiness or love, so I sabotaged the best thing I ever had. Everything was falling into place. I could see it all so clearly. And now that it was clear, now that I understood what I was close to losing, I could fix it.

I landed in Aruba the next day and Dennis was waiting. Walking toward him, I knew everything I'd done over the past months was wrong. I dropped my bag and threw my arms around his neck. He pulled me in close. Both of us cried. I realized that ever since I'd met him, however close we were, I'd always had one foot out the door. That was my MO. I didn't truly know how to stay in a relationship—a part of me was always looking for the next thing, the next step. I never felt like I could relax fully in one place. Hugging him at the airport, I felt his heart beat against mine. *I almost destroyed the best thing I ever had.* The thought was gut-wrenching, but somehow I knew then and there: we were going to be okay. I was going to make it all okay. He was the love of my life. Almost losing him brought an urgency to the relationship that I hadn't felt before. I knew now that there was nowhere else I wanted to be except with him. I had been awakened. I wasn't going anywhere, ever again. I was all in.

9

MOVE

Dennis and I settled back into our life in Aruba, healing from the past months of uncertainty. It started off shaky, but with time our relationship grew stronger. Before our challenges, whenever someone would joke about us having kids or getting married, I would squirm at the thought of that kind of commitment. But now, the idea didn't seem so ludicrous at all. Almost losing him woke me up, and brought me to some big realizations about my past and patterns that I'd carried with me into the present. Just because I'd moved a thousand miles away didn't mean that the issues I'd struggled with had disappeared all of a sudden. My fear of commitment was right there under the surface all along, and had it not been for the challenges Dennis and I faced that year I would have found other ways to self-sabotage. I knew now: I'd been lucky enough to find the love of my life. I was never going to risk losing him again.

Over the next year, I immersed myself in two things: my relationship and my career. Focusing on my yoga practice helped me heal and also gave me time to breathe new life into my teaching. On a whim, I had chosen the Instagram handle @yoga_girl and started gearing my social media presence more toward yoga—taking photos of beautiful poses and pairing them with musings about life and love. I tried not to filter my views but tell it the way it was. Not just the good, but the raw and difficult times as well. The more real I was, the more I revealed about my imperfect life, the more people related to me. I wasn't quite sure how it all happened, but more and more people were suddenly drawn to my account. As my online community grew from family and friends when I first started to thousands of people I didn't know, I began focusing a lot more energy toward social media. I was new to it—I'd just recently gotten my first-ever smartphone, years after all of my friends back in Sweden did, but I realized that it wasn't all that hard. I used the self-timer app on my phone to take photos of my yoga practice, and then shared them on Instagram paired with a caption about something I'd been pondering that day. In the beginning I wrote mostly about yoga, sharing tips and pieces of advice for people looking to begin a yoga practice. Soon questions started coming in and I did my best to answer them. "How far apart should you keep your feet in Downward-Facing Dog?" was a commonly asked one, or "What are some good yoga poses for me to help alleviate my back pain?" or "How can I find a teacher I resonate with?" As I became more comfortable sharing pieces of my life online, I started writing about more personal topics. After a while, baring my soul to complete strangers didn't feel odd at all. Every day I'd write about my search for balance, or self-love, or forgiveness. I realized that everything I'd ever felt, other people felt, too. I wasn't alone on this journey. It didn't take long before my community had grown so big that I couldn't keep up with answering all the questions anymore. When seemingly out of the blue I had reached 50,000 followers, I almost couldn't believe it. That was half the population of Aruba! I couldn't believe that so many people were interested in following my journey. I was grateful, and continued sharing my life through social media every day.

At the same time, my classes in Aruba filled up faster than I could post about them, and I was beginning to receive invitations to teach at studios in other countries. Dennis was in the midst of opening up a skate shop on the island, and we took a trip to Surf Expo in Orlando to place orders for the shop. One day when I was walking from one of the booths I saw a group of girls leaning in toward one another, whispering and pointing at me. I shook it off, thinking maybe they had me confused for someone, when I heard one of them say, "I swear! That's her, that's Yoga Girl!" I was mortified and picked up my pace to walk away as fast as I could. These people . . . They recognized me? From Instagram? That had never happened to me before, and for some reason, I felt ashamed. The way the girl had said it didn't sound positive—I felt exposed, looked at. A few hours later I saw the same group of girls, and this time they started walking my way. I took a deep breath, not knowing what to expect, when suddenly, one of them burst into tears. "Are you Yoga Girl? You are, right? I can't believe it! You have been such a huge inspiration to me—I found yoga thanks to you. It completely changed my life. Can we take a selfie?" I was stunned. I was an inspiration? What? I couldn't believe my ears. We took the photo, and as I put my arm around her shoulder I felt her shaking. "I'm sorry," she said. "I just can't believe it's you. Thank you for everything you do. Really." She hugged me tight, and before I knew it they were gone. Dennis looked at me like we'd just seen a UFO descend in front of us. He couldn't believe his ears either. "Whoa" he said. "That was kind of cool." "It was?" I asked. "Hell yes! She said you were the reason she found yoga, and that it changed her life! That's crazy! It means you're doing something good, babes." He hugged me.

It felt odd. How could I have impacted someone's life when I'd never even met them before? When a little later in the day I shared on Instagram that I was in Orlando, a few people commented asking if I could teach a class while I was there. Feeling empowered by my encounter at the expo, I decided to roll the dice and give it a try. What was the worst thing that could happen? I googled "Orlando + yoga studio" and proceeded to e-mail every yoga studio in the area, asking if any of them had space to host a class on short notice. Most didn't even bother to reply, and if they did it was with questions I didn't know how to answer. I didn't have a website, or any credentials, or a bio to send. When I told them I was planning to market the class through Instagram I was met with skepticism. This was 2012, and social media and yoga were a new combination. One studio in the Orlando suburbs wrote me back saying they'd be willing to open the space in exchange for a 50-50 split of the revenue. I said I thought maybe three or four people would come and that of course I'd be fine with any split! I was just looking forward to the opportunity to teach outside of Aruba. When it was time to drive to the class I was so nervous I had to ask Dennis to pull the car over because I was worried I might vomit. Thankfully I didn't, and when we made it to the studio I was met with a sight that made my jaw drop to the floor: there was a line from the studio entrance out into the street! *Was there some big event happening before my class?* I wondered. Walking in, all eyes turned to me. "Oh my God!" a woman said. "She's here!" The studio had a max capacity of thirty-seven people and more than fifty people had arrived, some having driven across Florida to be there. The woman in charge of checking people in was frantically trying to move things from the boutique so people could lay their mats down there, too. The biggest class I'd ever taught before that moment was probably around fifteen people. I hugged as many people as I could on the way in, and getting changed in the dressing room I thought to myself, *If you're going to panic, now is the time.* I didn't. Instead, I put my yoga pants on and stepped out into the room. When Dennis and I left the studio a few hours later, I was on cloud nine. I couldn't remember a single thing I'd just taught.

"It was great," Dennis said. "You were really, really great." I squeezed his hand. "Thanks," I said. "So . . . Do you think this is something we could do more of?" He looked at me. "Yeah. Definitely." That first class in Orlando sparked another, which sparked another, and another. A few months later Dennis and I embarked on a thirty-six-city tour across North America, teaching in as many places as we could get to. I got better at negotiating with studios (50-50 is a terrible deal!), and classes grew from fifty to eighty, and then up to a hundred people. My Instagram community was growing by the thousands every day. In a short time we'd created what seemed to be the perfect life—combining the skate shop in Aruba with traveling anywhere we wanted in the world, teaching yoga to pay our way. For us, it was an absolute dream.

It was on one of those trips that we ended up in Maui and one beautiful afternoon, Dennis took me up to the summit of the Haleakala volcano and proposed. We were above the clouds, watching the most breathtaking sunset either of us had ever seen, when suddenly he went down on one knee. My gut reaction wasn't pure joy, the way I'd imagined it, but actual panic—I had to take a deep breath and remind myself to stay put. I was so used to running, so used to self-sabotage, that I had to pause to bring myself back to the present moment. My whole life, all I'd known was separation, divorce, and loss. I didn't have a single person—parent or grandparent on either side of my family—who hadn't gotten divorced. I had no experience of what a solid commitment looked like and, in that moment, I had to remind myself of a couple of things: (1) You are not your past. You can break the cycle of struggle you were born into. (2) It is safe to love and be loved. Dennis isn't going anywhere. You went through the hard time and, still, he didn't waver. He's here to stay. Now it's up to you to decide if you are, too. Standing there on that mountaintop during one of the most important moments of my life, an old question I hadn't asked myself in a long time popped into my head: *What's the most loving thing to do here?* As I looked at Dennis, standing on one knee, tears in his eyes, the answer was resounding. The love of my life was in front of me, holding a ring. There was nothing to fear—there was only love. The answer came from deep inside my heart. Yes. Yes! A thousand times, yes.

I called my mom to tell her the news, but she already knew. Dennis had not only asked both of my parents for their blessings, but even had my grandmother's old wedding ring flown in from Europe. It was a merge of old and new—a piece of my past merging with my future wrapped around my ring finger. I remembered what the cacao shaman had told me: "Healing works both ways—it heals what's been before and what's yet to come." Wearing my grandmother's ring embodied that sentiment: I was closing wounds from long ago by choosing love here and now. It was beautiful. We spent the rest of the year feeling newly in love, over the moon with excitement. Looking at my life, I was in awe of how much had changed in such little time. In just a few years I'd gone from feeling depressed and stuck to being engaged to the love of my life, pursuing my greatest passion and traveling the world while doing so. How did I get so lucky?

When I hit a million followers on Instagram, Dennis and I celebrated with a glass of champagne—the size of the community was mind-blowing! It brought with it amazing opportunities to create anything we wanted. I was so grateful, but at the same time I missed the intimate privacy of our old lives. Getting recognized everywhere I went made me feel like I was always looked at but never seen. I started avoiding yoga studios and places I knew were filled with people who might want to approach me and soon the thought of another trip made me feel weary instead of excited. I knew I needed to slow down but kept saying yes to every opportunity that came my way.

After tons of back-to-back retreats and working for a year straight without a break, I flew to Costa Rica for the 2014

Envision Festival in February. By then, I was bone tired. Why did life feel as if it were getting away from me all of a sudden? By then, I was traveling every week for engagements away from home and my social media community had grown to the size of a small country. Every day I woke up to comments, questions, and sometimes judgments from people I didn't know. What had begun as an exciting way to see the world through my passion for yoga, however amazing, was also growing into a demanding and often stressful business. I needed a break before the festival and private time with my best friend.

Andrea was waiting at the airport when I landed in San José. I hadn't seen her since December, just two months earlier, when I'd asked her to be a bridesmaid in my wedding.

I'll never forget that day. I'd taught a retreat in the mountains above Dominical, and Andrea, who was new to yoga but intrigued, joined us for the week. Now the retreat had ended and we were watching the sunset on the beach, reminiscing about old times. We held hands walking out into the ocean, letting the golden rays of the sun warm our skin. I'd been waiting all day to broach the subject and it felt like the right moment.

"There's something I've been wanting to ask you," I said.

"What?"

"Okay, so don't freak out, but . . . Want to be my bridesmaid?"

Andrea's eyes flew open. "I thought you would never ask!" she cried. She waded over to me, smiling and laughing and hugging me so fiercely she pushed me over. A wave crashed over us and when we surfaced again she was laughing out loud.

I asked her, "Is that a yes?"

"*Yes!*" she squealed. "Oh my God! I'm going to be the best bridesmaid *ever*! I'll braid your hair. I'll take care of everything. But don't you go all bridezilla on me!"

"I'm already bridezilla." I laughed.

"We're going to *Sweden!*" she shrieked. "Sweden! Holy shit! This is going to be the best year!"

Now, picking me up at the airport two months later, Andrea hugged me again, but this time so tightly that I almost lost my breath. "Whoa!" I said. "You've missed me, huh?" She looked at me, her eyes serious. "I just felt like you needed a real hug. You've been so busy lately. We haven't spoken all week!" She was right. I wasn't taking as much time for my friends as I normally would, always with the excuse of teaching or traveling. I craved time with my bestie. We instantly settled back into our regular rhythm.

On my first night back, we drove to a little wine bar and spent the evening catching up. So much had happened in so little time. I was getting married, she had a new boyfriend. We were both in solid, committed places in our lives. She was studying hard at university, I was traveling the world teaching yoga. In a way, so many of our dreams had come true at the same time. I opened up about feeling exhausted, and when I did, Andrea said she'd been worried about me. "I know you're on this high, traveling the world, doing the social media thing," she said. "I just don't want you to rush through life. Your body is telling you something. You've got to slow down, love."

I knew she was right. I was suffering from neck pain on and off, and wasn't sleeping well. "I know I'm going somewhere, and it's somewhere good, but I feel like I've lost a piece

of myself," I said, suddenly tearing up. "And it's weird because
it's all such a huge blessing and I feel guilty complaining about
any of it. People stare at me all the time. I'm never alone, never
still anymore. I can't believe I'm saying it, but I miss what my
life was."

Andrea, ever the optimist, smiled. "But you have so much
freedom now," she said. "And influence! You can nudge people
to do the right thing. That's got to be pretty amazing, no? I
think you should just focus more on that—helping people.
You don't need to rush across the whole world for that. Slow
down. Figure out how you can be of true service. You won't feel
stressed when you're aligned with that place."

I knew she was right. I had such a beautiful life. I was about
to marry the love of my life. I got to travel the world doing
what I loved. I had been getting caught up in social media and
in building my business, but I didn't have a plan for any of it.
Everything had just snowballed and now I felt like I was losing
sight of what I was doing. I should just slow down and focus
on doing good things for the world. She always had a way of
making everything feel so easy.

After a few days together in San José, Andrea dropped
me off at the bus station for the four-hour ride south to the
tiny Pacific coast town of Uvita, where the festival was held.
Envision is a music, yoga, and art festival in the jungles of
Costa Rica. My friend Josh cofounded it years before and it
had grown from a gathering of friends to more than seven
thousand attendees over four days. I'd taught at the festival a
couple of times, but that year I was the yoga headliner. The
plan was that I would travel there a day ahead of Andrea while

she stayed behind to complete a project for her architectural studies.

The bus was filled with people who were headed to the event from the airport; mostly new age–looking girls in bikini tops and yoga pants, and men covered in Buddha-inspired tattoos. From the moment I stepped on, people began asking to take photos with me. Right away I felt exposed. Normally, I hid behind Dennis during these times, but I was alone and didn't quite know how to handle the attention. I put on a big smile the way I always did, and took selfies and chatted with everyone. As soon as I got a moment to myself I put on my headphones and listened to music for the rest of the trip.

Once we got there, I checked into a hostel. The room was small and bare, with two beds and a tiny bathroom. It looked clean enough and the air-conditioning worked, and that was all we really needed. The space felt cozier when I hung a few of my sarongs over the metal window frame.

It was late by the time I settled in, and my first class was early the next day. I took a photo of myself with the pink Costa Rican sky in the background and uploaded it to Instagram. I was feeling lonely and texted Andrea.

When are you coming?

She called right away, giggling. "Macha! Are you in our super-fancy hotel room? I've packed all my wigs and glitter and feathers and crazy clothing. We are going to have such a good time!" I couldn't help but smile. To Andrea, anything that wasn't camping was fancy. I'd convinced her to get a room because no matter how many times I tried to enjoy it, camping just wasn't for me. "Are you okay?" she asked. "Yes," I said. "I feel better now, just tired, and my neck hurts, and it's lonely here without you."

Andrea turned serious. "I've been telling you, it's not healthy to work this much," she said. "You have to pause. Remember why you're here." I paused. "And why am I here?" I asked, half joking. "To make the world a better place! Duh!" Andrea said. My eyes welled up and I was smiling again. "Now go to bed," she said. "I'm driving down first thing in the morning. Enjoy class! It's going to go great." I felt a lot better and fell asleep excited about our days ahead.

I woke up a little after sunrise. My neck pain was still bothering me, but I wouldn't let it bring me down. I dressed for class and waited for my friend Laura to pick me up and drive me to the festival. Whatever I'd been feeling the night before was gone. I was in Costa Rica, about to spend a week with my besties! Life was good!

Laura and I checked in to the festival and boarded the chicken truck (yep!) that served as a shuttle between parking and the festival grounds. When we got there, I realized how big my class was, despite the scorching sun. It was by far the biggest class at the event. I felt the butterflies in my stomach that I always felt before stepping onstage to lead people through a practice, but reminded myself that no one was there for me. I was merely the guide. We were all there for the same reason: to feel, breathe, and connect.

The class was lovely. By the end, I was feeling high on life and hugging everyone around me. Laura dropped me back at the hostel to wait for Andrea. As I wrapped myself in a towel after a shower, a bang came on the door. *"Machaaaaaaaa!!!!! I'm hooooommmmme!"* We both shrieked like schoolgirls when I opened the door. "We're here! All week! Just us!" she cried. Hugging her, I was so happy I almost started to cry. What was it about this week that was making me so emotional?

It was too hot to go back to the festival, so we decided to go in search of waterfalls. We called it waterfalling, *catarateando*. Andrea knew all of the hidden gems. We drove up the mountain, talking all the way. "Things are so good with Gabriel," she said. Gabriel was her boyfriend, a supersweet guy she'd been seeing for a long time now. "Wanna know a secret?" she said. "What?" "I want to have his babies!" she exclaimed with a big smile across her face.

I couldn't believe my ears. "Babies? Are you kidding?" I could see she was completely serious. "Maybe not right now," she said. "But not super long from now. I'm twenty-four! I feel ready. Almost." I didn't feel remotely ready for a baby, and the idea that Andrea was thinking about it made me feel like an outsider. Here she was, pondering a momentous life change, and I hadn't even known. "Does that sound so crazy?" she asked. It did. But it didn't. We weren't nineteen anymore! I was twenty-five, she was twenty-four. I was getting married, she was thinking about babies. We were growing up. How wild and beautiful life was.

Turning onto a dirt road, we came to a sudden stop. "This is it!" she exclaimed. We hiked to a clearing and there it was: a huge waterfall gushing down the side of a steep, vertical rock wall, a deep pool of blue at the bottom. It was breathtaking.

All alone, we took off our clothes and dove into the water. For the rest of the afternoon we swam, sunbathed on the rocks, and sang until our lungs hurt.

Driving back, I felt as if a weight had been lifted. My neck felt freer; my heart lighter. I sensed Andrea looking at me. "You look more like yourself already," she said. "Like myself? What do you mean?" I asked. "I don't know," she said. "You have a different look on your face these days. You're always busy. Always on your phone. I can tell by your voice when we talk that you need a break." I felt myself tear up again. She was right. I'd become so caught up in the idea of building a career, I'd lost sight of what I was doing it for. I missed the version of me that I was when I was with her.

Returning to the festival, we decided to set up a tent on the grounds in case we wanted to sleep on-site for any of the nights. The party went on all night, and the DJ of the sunrise set would hand off the microphone to the yoga teacher leading the first class of the day. Having a tent meant we had a place to keep our things, and a place to nap should we need it! We finished setting it up, took a yoga class, and then lounged on the grass afterward. Others joined us and we struck up a conversation about spirituality and what happens after you die. "For sure the cycle continues," Andrea said. "We're so connected to everything. Think about it. In nature, when a being dies, she becomes part of the earth, and in earth, new life grows. I'm happy I got to be who I am in this lifetime, but I don't feel nervous about dying. Whatever comes after this is bound to be pretty amazing, right? Just look around!" I looked around at the lush greenery. The sky was blue. Children laughed and played. Friends were engaged in conversation. Couples held hands, lounging in the grass. "Life," Andrea said. "It just unfolds the way it's supposed to. I don't think anything is a mistake." Andrea was young, but she was definitely an old soul.

We gathered our things and went back to the hotel for a quick shower and to get dressed up in full-on festival gear. I wore a skirt and moccasins, and a top that tied in a crisscross pattern across my back. Andrea wore a skirt and a bandeau top with her favorite vest over it. I tied feathers into my hair and we put sparkling gems around our eyes. We went all out, and at the end of it looked like we'd just stepped into the desert, about to attend Burning Man (which was sort of what we were going for). Andrea hung her leather pouch—my favorite one—around her waist. She got it during one of her trips to Guatemala—it's adorned with a jade gemstone in the front and is one of the most beautiful things I know. Whenever we saw each other I'd always borrow it. It's the perfect thing for nights out or when you're going dancing; you're perfectly free, no purse hung on your shoulder. "Okay, fine, you wear it!" she said, looking at me admiring it. "One day I'm going to give you a pouch just like this so you can stop trying to steal mine," she said, shoving me playfully. We walked out into the night, full of excitement.

Walking into the festival grounds at nighttime is a completely different experience. The festival area is big and spans across cow pastures and jungle, all the way to the beach and the ocean. In the daytime there are lectures on everything from healthy eating to farming to sustainable living to medicinal herbs. There is a big village area with food and vendors and little stalls selling jewelry and clothing and crystals, a kids' area with fun activities for children, a Red Tent (gatherings specific to women and womb wisdom). Basically all the new age things you could ever imagine. It's beautiful! At night, the energy changes from family, yoga, and surf to deep tribal dance party. The stages are built in bamboo and all boast different DJs and artists. Scattered around the grounds are bars serving elixirs and juices, and everywhere you go you see people dancing, dancing, dancing. That's the main part of the festival: the music. You hear the beat from miles away. Andrea and I ran through the festival gates filled with anticipation for the night ahead. We skipped the bar and went straight to the main stage to catch a reggae band we'd always loved. Andrea burst through the crowd and started dancing. Dancing was her thing—it was amazing just to watch. She let the music move through her in a way that was almost childlike; she wasn't thinking about dancing, or what she looked like, or if anyone was watching . . . she just danced. She became the dance—maybe the dance danced through her. It's hard for me to explain. I was always an awkward dancer, and every time I was in a festival setting it took me a little while to ease into the music, to release my inhibitions, to fully let go. I always felt judged, or looked at—which I know wasn't the case. It just always took me a little while to get into my body. I wanted to feel as free as Andrea looked the second she started moving with the music: eyes closed, hips swaying, hair across her face. I felt stiff in comparison. For her, dancing was meditation, the way yoga asana was for me. A few songs in I felt myself relaxing a bit more, easing my way in. If I tapped into my breath and focused on the feeling, I could sense the beat of the music vibrating in my heart. I was lost in the music, too. We danced and danced. Reggae became electronica, which became dance music; it didn't matter. There is rhythm in everything and I was one with it. Suddenly the music stopped—the main stage acts were over. We'd been dancing for hours and hadn't had a sip of water. Realizing how thirsty we were, we wobbled over to the village area, high on music. I bought us two kombuchas and some food—tacos and a veggie burrito—and we sat down in the grass.

I was soaked in sweat but in the best way. We ate in silence—food had never tasted so good. The kombucha was ice-cold. I looked up at Andrea. She was smiling to herself, picking coleslaw and black beans from her plate. It struck me: We hadn't spoken a word in hours. We didn't have to. There was nothing to say. "Hey," I said. "What?" she said. "You're my best friend, you know that?" She laughed. "Duh. I was just thinking, the fact that we don't have to talk all the time is amazing. I don't know anyone else I can just be silent with and not have it be weird." I smiled. We spent the rest of the night dancing. Around three in the morning we made our way to a fire circle in a quiet area of the festival. The sky was bright with stars, the air smelling of smoke. Someone played a soft, rhythmic beat on a drum. I leaned up against a tree trunk and must have fallen asleep, because when I opened my eyes the circle was smaller, Andrea sitting in the middle, talking. She was deep in conversation with someone about ayahuasca and was sharing her experience with the psychedelic vine with the group. I realized it was a story I had never heard before. It was strange, hearing her telling a story I didn't know. It was similar to hearing her say she wanted to have babies—I felt like I was on the outside looking in. Our bond was so strong that it always surprised me to hear of things I didn't know; but of course that was the case. We lived in two different countries. We had an ocean between us, different lives that didn't involve talking every single day. It made me sad and happy at the same time. The number of friends like that, whom I could connect with at any time and just pick up where we left off . . . I could count them on a few fingers. Andrea saw that I was awake and came over to sit by my side. "When did you do that ayahuasca ceremony?" I asked. "Last year!" she said. "As I was telling the story I realized I never told you—isn't that weird?" "It's like how you have these pieces of your life now that I know nothing about. Like that story you told me at the waterfall about opening a studio; I've never even heard you mention that before and it's this big huge dream? It's crazy!" I was baffled by how much we thought alike. "Do you ever miss Costa Rica? Like, you'd want to move back here?" I thought about it. "Miss it? Yes. Want to move back? No." I looked up at the sky. "I guess this is what growing up is like," I said. "Having people you love in different places." "Yup. But you want to know the good part about that? We get to travel! *Like to Sweden!!* I can't believe we're going to Sweden. You're getting married. It's nuts!" I'd almost forgotten about that. My whole life was so busy—work, travel, teaching, social media—I was squeezing in wedding planning as best I could on the side. "We are going to Sweden! And I'm getting married! Holy shit. It's all so surreal." Andrea and I had traveled together but only to Colombia, Miami, and around Costa

Rica. Sweden was a big deal. I held back a yawn. "Wanna go watch the sunrise from the beach?" "Always!" We grabbed a big blanket from the tent and headed over to the shore. It was still dark but there was a hint of golden light coming from the jungle. We spread the blanket out in a quiet place and sat down. With the sand beneath me and the energy of the sun rising, I felt an electric energy rising within me. I closed my eyes and together we sat like that, in silence, in meditation, until we felt the first rays of the sun on our faces. I opened my eyes and realized my cheeks hurt—I'd been smiling the whole time. Andrea still had her eyes closed. Her gray mala beads were in her hands. I stood up. "I wish I had my bathing suit!" I said. "It would be so nice to take a swim right now." Andrea opened her eyes. "Who needs one?" she said, and pulled her shirt over her head. For the shortest moment, I hesitated. Naked? Here? There were people around! Not super close, but still. It wasn't some secluded waterfall, it was the beach right by the festival. More and more people were spilling onto the beach to watch the sun come up. Andrea was already halfway to the water. *Fuck it*, I thought. I took a deep breath, took my clothes off, and followed her.

There is something truly awesome about waking up in your hostel room after a full night out without even the hint of a hangover. After our swim in the morning, we left the festival and headed back to our hostel. Thanks to the air-conditioned room, we'd gotten a whole seven hours of sleep. We met up with Laura for breakfast: gallo pinto (Costa Rican rice and beans) with toast, fresh tomato, and avocado. And hot sauce. My favorite. We went on and on about the night before with Laura, how we danced all night, the fire, the people, the sunrise . . . And this was only our first full festival day! Laura never came to the festival at night; the daytime activities were more her thing. We decided to find another waterfall and Laura joined us. It required a bit of a hike and also a swim to get to where we were going, but once we got there . . . it was magical. We took a photo in front of the waterfall with our tops off, shrieking with joy. Laura dropped us off at the hostel to get ready for another night of wild dancing. Andrea decided to wear her blue wig and I put on my favorite dress. We drank a beer in the room, listening to Toploader's "Dancing in the Moonlight" on repeat. Andrea put on a show and I caught it on my phone and sent it to Gabriel. He laughed—"Make sure you take care of her! That wig always means trouble!" This night of the festival came with some amazing acts. We did a bit of shopping in the village area—I got braids to clip into my hair and found a supercute green skirt. Andrea, true to her aversion to shopping—spent an entire hour contemplating whether to get the same skirt in black, and it took walking back and forth over and over and trying it on a hundred times before she decided to get it. "It's twenty bucks!" I said. "*Just get it!!!*" "But think of all the things I can do with twenty bucks!" she said. "I could get us a full dinner! For two! Or if we go to that kind of crappy place on the corner in Dominical it's a dinner for four! *A full couples dinner*. Dude. No. I can't buy it." She put it back. "If you ever take us to that place for couples dinner I will buy that skirt just so I can strangle you with it. That place is the worst!" She laughed. "Okay, fine. I guess I do like it a lot. I'll take it." She paid and then spent another hour asking me again and again if it was the right purchase. She was funny like that—super spontaneous and in the moment about everything, except spending money. She hated to shop. I, on the other hand, did not have this problem. Money seemed to run away from me—a skirt here, a pair of earrings there . . . I never thought much about money. Sometimes it felt like I had a lot of it. Sometimes I felt flat broke. I wasn't attached to either side, but I wish I had a little more patience and that I wasn't so quick to spend on a whim.

An amazing electronica band was playing that night, so after Andrea finally put on her new skirt we went over to dance. On our way there we ran into Luigi! Luigi, our Luigi. Luigi was like a brother to us, one of the pieces in our close-knit puzzle. Luigi and I dated briefly years earlier and when things ended between us, we became close friends. When me, Andrea, Josh, and Luigi hung out together we always called it "family time" because that's what we were—family. Luigi and Andrea had become super close since I'd left the country and saw each other almost every day. We hadn't seen him at the festival at all. He was on the production team and was always crazy busy the week of. "Macha! Loca! If it isn't my favorite people in the whole wide world!" He scooped us both up in a big bear hug. "Topsy!!" I said, using my favorite nickname for him. "We've missed you. Come dance with us." "Okay, for a little, but I have to head backstage and deal with something. And we have sound check in thirty minutes. Make sure you are at the Sol Stage on time!" Luigi was in a band, Patterns, that was becoming increasingly famous in Central and South America. They had just opened for Depeche Mode and their set was highly anticipated at the festival. We danced and hugged, and a second later, Luigi was gone. "Tss," Andrea said. "Our little rock star. He's too famous for us now." As she said that, someone came up and asked to take a photo with me. It was a fairly frequent thing; every few minutes someone would come up to say hi. I took the photo and turned back to Andrea. "Actually—the both of you! I have this rock-star guy to my left and this yoga girl to my right. Who knew my besties would become so famous and important." She pouted. "He better bring us along when he's a world-famous artist—and you better bring us along when . . ." I tried to finish the sentence for her: "When . . . what? I'm still the same person!" She laughed. "I don't know. I feel like you are going somewhere that's bigger than this. Time will tell," she said. I hugged her. "Okay, now stop talking shit so we can enjoy the show!" We turned back to the stage and danced. We met so many people that night: fire dancers, a shaman who gave us cacao from a big pot, a guy dressed only in body paint . . . We kept finding ourselves entrenched in deep conversation about life with the strangest characters I could think of. When we danced there was something almost electric about it; I'm pretty sure it was Andrea—people would just stop and stare when they saw her, and then come talk to us. Later in the evening we were getting ready to see a band we'd heard good things about but never seen before: Nahko and Medicine for the People, and before that, the Human Experience. At the village getting food, I saw that Andrea looked tired. She yawned. "I think I need a catnap," she said. "Wanna go to the tent and rest a little?" I didn't want to miss the first act but I didn't mind taking a break so Andrea could rest. Festival nights were like that; they went on for so long, sometimes you just needed a little break in the middle. "Yes, but you stay! I know you want to see the next act. Go enjoy and let's meet backstage, by the stairs on the right side, in an hour?" "Sure," I said. "But promise you will be there! Set an alarm on your phone!" "Yes, Mom," she said, rolling her eyes. "One hour sharp." We parted ways; I headed back to the stage and Andrea walked toward the tent that we'd set up but never once slept in.

The Human Experience was amazing—unbelievable. I felt none of the insecurity or awkwardness of the first night but danced freely, by myself in a huge crowd of people, to every single song. I kept track of the time and made sure to be in the right place when it was time to meet Andrea, but she wasn't there. She was always a little late so I didn't think much of it. Twenty minutes later the set was over, but still no Andrea. They were setting up for the next band and I was a little bit in the way, so I decided to head over to the tent to wake her up. When I got there, it was empty. No sign of her having been there at all. I started getting a little worried and went to all our regular places—the food areas, the shop where she'd agonized about the skirt (wouldn't be surprised if I found her back there, returning it!)—and called her about a thousand times. No answer. After looking absolutely everywhere, I heard them announcing Nahko on the main stage and felt a strong pull to go back. The one place she'd go back to if we lost each other would be the last place we decided to link up, right? Andrea wasn't there, but I decided to watch the show from that spot, up close. I wasn't in the crowd but almost onstage, to the right of the artists. I didn't have any big expectations for the show and was mostly worried about Andrea—where could she be?—but when the music started . . . something happened to me. Nahko started singing and all of time stopped. There was something about the music, the lyrics, the beat, the message, all of it together that just blew my heart wide open. For the entire length of the set I stood almost frozen. "I believe in the good things coming, coming, coming, coming," he sang. "Everything's already all right always all right always all right." It was, hands down, the most powerful concert experience I'd ever had. I was all alone, one with the music. A photographer took a photo of me in that very moment—she e-mailed it to me later—and my entire face is beaming. It's one of my favorite photos I have of myself.

The show ended and it wasn't until I touched my hands to my face that I realized I was crying. I left floating. Suddenly I heard "Macha!!! I'm here!" and I looked up—Andrea was walking toward me. She had a blanket wrapped around her shoulders and looked sleepy. "*Where have you been??*" I said. "I looked everywhere!" She hugged me. "Sorry, sorry. The tent was too hot so I went to go sleep in the car with the windows down. My phone died so the alarm didn't go off." "I was so worried!" I said. "Don't worry about me, silly. Even when you think I'm far away I'm always nearby. I'm always here."

She said so many things like that that week—things I would reflect on for years afterward. We went to the hostel and I told her about everything she'd missed—the best show of all time! At the hostel I played her the song "Black as Night" and we lay on the bed, listening to it on repeat. I found a YouTube clip of an acoustic, live version of the song. We probably listened to it twenty times before we went to bed.

The next day we got to the festival early for yoga and spent the whole day there. We swam, listened to music, lounged in the grass, and just talked and talked and talked. There was a big, giant-sized dream catcher made of rope hung up between palm trees over one of the stages and we climbed up into it, dangling our feet from up in the air. "Can you believe that in only three months we are flying to Sweden? It's so wild," she said. "It's mine and Gabriel's biggest trip together for sure. And I'm finally going to meet the other bridesmaids! I can't believe it's in a *castle*. Whoa. What are all the Costa Rican hippies going to do in a castle?? I can't wait to dance my butt off." I could imagine it already; getting ready, putting our dresses on, doing one another's hair, me nervous about walking down the aisle . . . Actually, just thinking about it made me nervous. "You have to calm me down in case I start panicking," I said. Andrea started laughing. "You're not gonna panic! You might turn into Bridezilla, but you're not going to panic. It's Dennis. It's perfect." I pushed her lovingly. "I know. And I'm not going to be Bridezilla!" "You sort of are already, just a tiny bit . . ." She laughed. "But in a good way! It wouldn't be you if you didn't obsess about all the details being perfect." We laughed. I did want everything perfect and had had many a call with the vendors to alter things along the way. Suddenly she got serious. She looked at me. "Listen. I am so unbelievably proud of you. I don't think I say it enough." "Stop it," I said. "I haven't done anything special." "No—I mean it. You're building this whole life, with Dennis, you're creating something that's so beautiful. And I'm so proud to have you in my life. I love you so much." She started tearing up. "Why do you have to be so sappy! You're making me cry!" I said. "I mean it. Whatever happens, wherever we end up . . . I want you to know that. That I love you so much." We hugged and stayed like that, holding each other, for a long time.

"Oh my god—look!" Andrea exclaimed. "It's your music man!" She pointed, and walking toward us was Nahko, the singer from the show the night before. As he walked below us she reached down and touched his head. "Hey, music man! Up here!" He looked up and smiled. "Hey! What's up! It's a beautiful day, right?" "It sure is," she said. He waved and walked on. "I'm bummed I missed that show! He seems like a cool dude. Oh well. You gotta learn how to do some things without me." She leaned her head on my shoulder. I looked up at the sky. It was a beautiful, beautiful day.

You gotta learn how to do some things without me. I'd think about that one, too.

After a week together, we drove to the airport, listening to music and trying to come down from the high of our time at the festival. The closer we got to San José, the sadder I felt. *I'd said good-bye to Andrea so many times before, so why was this time so hard?* I wondered.

Pulling into the airport, I started to cry. It was the combination of so many things: the incredible week we'd just had, almost getting married, leaving my best friend . . . so much emotion wrapped up in one moment. Andrea squeezed my hand. "I know," she said. Tears were streaming down her face, too. "I know." We got out of the car and I pulled my suitcase from the trunk. "I don't want to go," I said. "I don't want you to go either," she said. We hugged, and as she let me go, I felt her hand go to my purse. I saw that she had left an envelope. "I didn't want you to see it!" She laughed through her tears. "I wanted it to be one of those things you randomly find when you're unpacking and then you call me and we smile about it together." I smiled. "You have to get better at your sneaking," I said. "Don't read it now," she said. "Read it on the plane or whenever you miss me." "Okay," I said. "I love you, gemela." Andrea turned to look at me one last time before she stepped back into the car. "I love you, too," she said. Then she was gone.

Sadness filled my heart. I cried silent tears through customs, and all the way into the plane. Why was I feeling so sad? I was going to see her in just a few months! Reaching into my purse for a tissue, my hand felt the envelope. As the plane took off, I opened it. It was a card. On the cover was a painting of a large spiral, framed by forests on both sides, with a shell sitting on the shore. As I studied it, the spiral seemed to move in both directions at the same time, an optical illusion. Transfixed, I opened it.

Always remember
Your light, your feet
In the sand
Your EARTH

Take care of that beautiful soul & body
I love you machita

For all the roads we have walked
And all the roads left to walk.

I love you.
Andre <3 Macha
Envision 2014

As I read Andrea's words, my sadness shifted. *I have such a beautiful life*, I thought. In just a few months I would walk down the aisle to marry the man of my dreams, and my best friend would be by my side. Gratitude washed into the space where the sadness had been. I posted a photo of the card on social media with a message:

On a plane, crying. Jetlag tired, festival smelly, rainforest dirty. But covered in glitter. And feathers. And love. Happy heart. Blessed with the best friend anybody could ever ask for. Gracias gemela por el amor infinito. Por todos los caminos recorridos y los que faltan por recorrer.

10

PROCESS

Two weeks later I was lying in a hospital bed listening to that incomprehensible word echoing in the back of my head. *Falleció.* Andrea was gone. I'd lost my best friend. Life, as I knew it, was over.

It didn't make sense. Nothing made sense. Our time at the festival had been so unbelievably beautiful—I'd just hugged her a moment ago, and now they were telling me she was dead? That she was gone? It couldn't be. I was in a state of shock, dialing her number again and again, waiting for her to pick up and tell me it was all some terrible mistake.

I felt like I was moving through a fog. I couldn't stand up straight after the surgery I'd just had and my whole body ached, but nothing could compare to the feeling of despair I felt in my chest. It was slowly suffocating me. I lost the ability to function altogether and stopped eating and sleeping. Nothing mattered anymore. After a few days all I wanted was to be left alone because I knew that whenever I picked up the phone to dial Andrea's number, everyone looked at me like I was crazy. They were all expecting me to understand, for it to sink in, but I refused to accept it as truth. How could the most alive person I'd ever known suddenly be dead? There was no way. I called her, again and again, hoping she would pick up, hoping she would answer and tell me it was all just a dream. She never did. I had so many questions. Andrea had been at a concert by the beach on the night of the crash. She and her boyfriend, Gabriel, had driven there separately. She was a few minutes ahead of him on the way back home. He came upon a traffic jam. People ahead of him had stepped out of their cars, trying to see what was going on. He heard someone say something about a car accident. "A bad one. A truck and an SUV." Andrea drove an SUV. Gabriel left his car, the keys dangling in the ignition, and ran. He saw Andrea's silver Toyota turned upside down, demolished. When he got to her she was still breathing.

He rode with her in the ambulance to the closest hospital but it wasn't equipped to treat the extent of her wounds. They had to turn around and go to San José. When they finally got there, the ER resident in charge turned them away. They were out of the hospital's jurisdiction, he'd said. The "right" hospital was thirty minutes away. In the papers afterward they called it "the ride of death." The whole country would come to know of Andrea's accident and all the mistakes that were made by medical professionals along the way. She was taken straight into surgery when they finally got to a hospital that would take her in. She was bleeding internally. Hours had passed since the accident. They performed surgery on her abdomen to stop the bleeding. In another country, at the same time, I was writhing with stomach pain. Andrea had two heart attacks. Her body couldn't take it anymore. It seemed as if no one knew all the details of what exactly had happened, so I did my best to piece things together.

At first it seemed that Andrea had ended up in oncoming traffic, which didn't make sense. She never used her phone while driving. She was a good driver and she'd driven that road so many times. Had she been looking for something and gotten distracted? Did she fall asleep? Was it possible that the extra minutes between hospitals made the difference between life and death? Later we found out it wasn't she who ended up in oncoming traffic, but the truck. She never had a chance. In the end, did it matter? She was dead. I felt like I died with her.

The last time we were together, Andrea had told me, "Don't worry, macha. Even when I'm far away I'm always nearby." Then why couldn't I feel her? Why hadn't she given me a sign that she was near? Why had she lied?

A few days after my surgery, I was released from the hospital in Bonaire. My body was healing. My heart was not.

I posted a photo of Andrea and me on Instagram with a message for her. I wanted the whole world to know that we lost an angel and that my heart was broken. A part of me thought that if I spoke the words out loud, if I wrote them down for the world to see, it would help me understand that it was all actually real. That it wasn't a dream. The time we spent together last time I saw you and the conversations leading up to your death were so intense, so full of love, I'm wondering now: why didn't I see this coming? You left me more voice messages than you ever have, just telling me you love me. You hid letters in my suitcase.

You hugged me so tight. Why didn't you let me know those were the last days? Why didn't you let me say good-bye?

Andrea was cremated in Costa Rica but I was stuck in Bonaire, waiting for the doctor to give me permission to fly. I still couldn't walk or bend forward or stand up straight. All I wanted was to lie in bed under the covers with the curtains drawn, but Dennis wouldn't let me. Every day, he opened up the drapes and carried me out of bed and held me under the shower. One day he even shaved my legs. "If you want her to talk to you, go sit by the ocean," he said one morning. "Go at sunrise and meditate with the wisdom we all know you have inside. Don't lie here in the dark. She is in the light, so go where there is light and speak to her." I knew he was right, but the dark was so comforting. And what if I tried to reach her but she didn't answer? Or what if she did? Then everything would be real and I preferred that it weren't. Except I was starting to understand that it was.

Many of our friends flew in to be with us. I had an outpouring of support flooding my way but I felt none of it. The first sign of light came a few days later. After everyone had left the house we were renting I went with my friend Rose to sit on the dock in the sunshine. She swam and I lay on a towel. A feeling overtook me. I wanted to be naked—to shed some of the heavy layers weighing me down. But there were people on the island, so how did I dare strip down to nothing? I thought to myself, *What would Andrea do? Andrea wouldn't give one gram of a fuck.* Andrea would say, "If you need to be free, you need to be free!" So I took it all off, ran screaming across the pier in all my glory, and threw myself into the ocean. When I came up to the surface there was light glittering all around me. It was so special—like I was swimming in a pool of it. I'd never seen light glistening across the ocean in that way before. The water was so soft, so clear, so comforting. I called out to Rose, "*Hey!*" "What?" she asked. "*I feel something!*" I shouted. "That's good!" she said. I felt something and that was not nothing. Afterward I sat down on the pier and opened to the first page of a brand-new notebook. At the top of the page I wrote: "To the light that glitters across the ocean as the sun sets." Out of me poured a love letter to Andrea. I sat there for more than an hour, writing to her. When I finished I felt a strange sense of calm in my heart. I realized there were many ways to talk to her. The light would show me the way. If only it would last; but grief doesn't work that way. The moment dissipated as quickly as it came and I fell back into the darkness.

I started listening to the song "Black as Night" by Nahko and Medicine for the People again. Andrea and I had listened to the song over and over during the Envision Festival. It was our most recent anthem. Now it became my obsession. I listened to it on repeat. "I believe in the good things coming, coming, coming, coming." I cried with the lyrics because I so badly wanted them to be true. I realized I was stuck in the in-between. I was still alive, but I'd lost the ability to be happy. I felt cold. Dead. Empty. I was supposed to be planning my wedding, but the thought of life returning to any degree of normal was too far away to grasp. I didn't know what I was looking for. All I knew was that my heart was in San José and I needed to get there.

As soon as I was cleared to travel, Dennis booked the

flight to Costa Rica. When we boarded the plane, I was in such an emotional spiral that another passenger asked the flight attendant to help me. I was hyperventilating and crying. They brought me water to drink, and tissues to wipe my tears, because what else could they do?

We arrived in San José and grabbed a taxi to Andrea's house, where her whole family was waiting. Standing at the front door, I froze. Everyone was inside: Her mom, Doña Patri; her sister, Juli; her aunt and cousins; and Gabriel, her boyfriend. *How will I face them?* I wondered. I wasn't sure I could. I looked at Dennis, standing on the sidewalk, holding Ringo in his arms. I could see that he, too, was terrified. "Are you ready?" he asked. "No," I said. He hugged me. "You'll feel close to her here," he said. I opened the door.

Just inside was a table with flowers, a lit candle, and Andrea's picture. She was wearing a scarf and smiling. Andrea's mom saw me first and her jaw dropped. She looked as if she'd seen a ghost. She grabbed me and held me and I began to sob. *This is so wrong*, I thought. I wanted to comfort her, not the other way around. We held each other for a few minutes before she spoke. "I forgot how much you look like her," she said. "For a moment, it was like she just walked through the door." Her eyes were red and her skin pale. I greeted the others, and someone handed me a plate of food. That's how it always was at Andrea's house. It felt the same this time—except she wasn't there, so nothing was the same. Everyone was talking and I felt a hand on my shoulder. When I turned around, Gabriel was standing there. His face was so tense I barely recognized him.

We hugged for a long time. *How would he get through this?* I wondered. How would any of us?

Dennis and I slept in Andrea's bed. That night I woke up crying from a terrible nightmare. I dreamt we were all staying in a huge house for Andrea's funeral. It was so full of people I couldn't find a place to sit. As I stood there, looking for somewhere to rest my legs, a family with a small baby approached me to say they were there for Ringo. I didn't understand. Why Ringo? I asked. "Because you're giving him to us, and we're taking him," they said. "This was decided months ago." I turned to Dennis in a panic. "Who decided this?" I asked. "You did," he replied. And then they took Ringo and he was gone. The dream ended with me screaming for him to come back. When I awakened, I knew. Ringo was Andrea, but my mind still couldn't process it. I couldn't let go.

On our second night, Doña Patri asked me to sleep at Andrea's house.

No one had slept there since the accident, but she insisted I go. "I think she would have wanted that," she said. "Go sleep there tonight. See if she is there. See if you feel her. I feel so near her when you are here. Go stay in her space. Please."

We made plans for Gabriel to take me; Dennis would meet up with us later.

Andrea loved her house. It was tiny but beautiful, nestled in the jungle on a mountaintop above San José. Gabriel's knuckles were white as we drove. Sitting in the passenger seat,

I noticed his car smelled really bad. Gabriel worked with sustainable fishing projects so I assumed there were fishing nets or equipment or something in the car.

"What is that smell?" I finally asked.

He was quiet. "It's her," he said after a moment of silence.

"What do you mean, her?" I asked.

"It's Andrea."

"I don't understand."

"Her things," he said. "From the accident. They had to cut her dress open to operate. It's covered in blood. They put it in a bag with her sweater and all of her bracelets and all her other things."

"And you have it . . . here? In the car?"

"I didn't know what to do with it."

We drove on in silence.

Andrea's house looked exactly the way I remembered it. Why did I think it would be any different? I handed Gabriel the keys, thinking he should be the first one in. When he pushed the door open, I saw his hands shake. We stepped inside. Everything was there except Andrea: the rug on the floor, the little couch by the window, dishes in the kitchen sink—a few glasses, a teacup. *We cooked in that kitchen just days ago*, I thought. She'd made a smoothie and I laughed at her because it came out almost black. "What the hell did you put in here?" I laughed. "Are you trying to poison me?" She threw a kitchen towel at my head. "It's good for you! Just drink it!" I smiled faintly at the memory. How could it be that she was just here? And now she was gone.

It was getting hard to breathe. I opened the kitchen door to let in some air. "Do you want to go upstairs?" I asked Gabriel. He was white as a ghost. "I can't do it," he said. We were quiet for a while. I could tell he was itching to leave. "Do you want to get the bag with her things?" I asked.

Gabriel went out to the car and came back carrying a plastic bag marked "Medical Waste." "Let's do this outside," I said. We walked out to the garden. Looking at the bag in front of me, I felt as if I were in some alternate universe. Surely this wasn't real. I took a deep breath, opened the bag, and reached my hand inside. I grasped something and I pulled a long piece of fabric from the bag. It was Andrea's dress, a light gray dress stained black with dried blood. Now my hands were the ones shaking. Slowly, I emptied the rest of the bag. Everything she wore on the day of the accident was there. Her dress, a sweater, some jewelry. It was all covered in blood. The last thing was her favorite necklace, a string of grayish-blue pearls that hung all the way down past her belly button. She loved that necklace—at Envision she wore it almost every day. The necklace was broken and the pearls lay scattered in the bottom of the bag. I took them out, one by one, and placed them on a log in the corner of the garden.

Gabriel couldn't take anymore.

"I have to go," he said. "Dennis is probably on his way. Are you okay to stay on your own?"

Standing in Andrea's garden brought me a strange sense of calm.

"Are *you* okay?" I asked.

Gabriel looked at me but didn't answer my question. "I'll call you later," he said.

Gabriel left and I wandered back into the house. By then, the sky was turning a dusty yellow, bathing the kitchen in a gentle light. I decided to go upstairs. The stairs creaked under my weight. At the top of the staircase was Andrea's altar, with her favorite crystals, stones, and gems. She would sit by the altar every day to meditate. I felt pulled to it like a magnet as I walked past and into her bedroom.

The first thing that struck me when I walked into her room was how tidy it was. Everything was neatly organized and clean, and the bed was made with her favorite throw across the duvet. I'd never seen Andrea's house so clean. She was a messy person, even messier than me. In the bathroom, her Envision Festival bracelet hung over a ledge by the shower. Mine was still on my wrist. I reached into the shower, took the bracelet, and held it against my own. Just as I did, I heard a car pull up. Dennis and Ringo were outside.

The three of us settled into Andrea's house. As the sun set we cooked dinner. I couldn't bring myself to touch the dishes in the sink; her dishes, the ones she had used before she left home for the last time. I was too afraid to disrupt the things that she last touched, and everything that still echoed with remembrances of her. Of course, everything did. The house vibrated with her energy. A thought crossed my mind: I know her things are just objects. But these things—the dishes she left in the sink before getting in the car and heading to the beach—they feel so recent. I can imagine her having her tea and leaving the cup before rushing out the door. She probably thought she'd do the dishes when she got back. But she never came back. And now I'm here, trying to avoid a dish that's not mine to clean.

At the dinner table I sat in Andrea's chair. Dennis sat in the one I normally used. We finished our meal and Dennis said he was ready for bed. It had been a long day. I almost stopped him when he headed into the shower. *Wait! That's her shower. She was the last one to shower there.* It felt wrong for him to use it. She was the last one to step on those tiles and turn the hot-water knob. I felt as if Dennis touching it would break the connection to her, but I decided not to say anything. I knew I was being crazy. Not stepping into Andrea's shower was not going to bring her back. Trying to keep her house frozen in time wouldn't either. Dennis kissed me good night and took Ringo into the bedroom with him. I was happy he turned in early because a part of me wanted to sit alone by Andrea's altar and just breathe. *If I could only quiet my mind, maybe I'd be able to feel her*, I thought. *What if I can't?*

Several candleholders were set up on the windowsill and half-burnt candles sat on the altar. I looked around the room for matches but couldn't find any. *With all of the candles scattered around, there have to be matches in the house*, I thought. I checked everywhere. Absolutely everywhere. In all of the kitchen drawers. On the coffee table by the sofa. On every damn shelf. I knew there must be boxes of matches around! Andrea was always burning candles and incense and palo santo. She even occasionally smoked tobacco from a pipe, Native American style. *Where are the goddamn matches? All I want to do is sit by this altar and pray!* I couldn't pray without candles! After frantically looking in every corner of the house with no luck, something inside of me snapped. Tears burned in my eyes. "*Andrea!*" I screamed out loud. "*Where are the fucking matches?*"

The moment the words left my mouth I felt a force turn my head to the left. It was extremely strange because I wasn't the one turning my head; someone turned my head for me, forcefully. My eyes landed on a picture frame on a shelf—a photo of Osho. My photo. How had I not noticed it before? Osho was one of my spiritual teachers and someone whose teachings had deeply impacted my life. When I was living in Dominical, my mom brought a framed photo of Osho when she came to visit me, which I hung by my altar. When I moved to Aruba I left most of my things behind, including the Osho picture. I had no idea Andrea had taken it and kept it in her house. Gabriel told me later it had been there for so many years—I'd just never noticed it before. Lowering my gaze slightly, I saw something that almost made my heart jump out of my chest. A box of matches was sitting there, leaning against the picture frame. I opened it. There was one single match inside. I dropped to my knees in tears, clutching the matchbox to my heart. Andrea's presence was so strong I could almost feel her arms around me. I was overcome with a sense of calm.

Standing in front of the altar, I realized that I didn't have to sit in formal meditation to feel Andrea. I didn't need candles, or an altar, or special moments. She was there, with me. All the time.

I moved past the altar and opened the door to the bedroom. There was a low cabinet on the floor and I spotted a candle sitting by some crystals next to Andrea's mala beads. I sat down to light the candle, realizing I only had one chance to make it work. I struck the match along the side of the matchbox. After lighting the candle, I blew out the match but dropped it while the tip was still a golden amber color. It had disappeared under the cabinet. *Crap*, I thought. Not only was the match still hot, I wanted to take it home with me. It was my first real connection to Andrea since she died. I had to retrieve it.

I lay on the floor and reached my arm under the cabinet to grab the match. When I did, I felt something else there. I pulled it out: a tiny statue of Mary Magdalene. Andrea had found her way back to her Catholic religion in the past year. We had talked about it at Envision a few weeks earlier. The concept of religion had always been foreign to me. Sweden is the most nonreligious country in the world, and I had no relationship to a church, Jesus, or the Bible. Andrea told me stories about Mary Magdalene, "the forgotten goddess." She was proud that she had gotten back to the church; it had brought her closer to her mom. "I still prefer to meditate and sit in circle over going to church, but I'm starting to appreciate where I've come from," she'd told me.

Looking at the figurine in my hand, remembering our conversation from a few weeks earlier, I felt the same pull as I had when my head turned toward the picture of Osho. This time, though, my hand was being pulled farther under the cabinet. *There is something else there*, I thought.

I lengthened my reach and my hand grasped a box. I pulled it out. It was green cardboard, beautifully adorned with flowers and doodles, and far too pretty to be hidden. My hands trembled as I opened the lid. It took a minute for me to figure out what I was looking at. It was my handwriting. Displayed neatly at the top of the box was our wedding invitation with Andrea's name written on the envelope. Andrea had guided me there.

Seeing our wedding invitation, I started to cry again and now I couldn't stop. As I lay on the floor, clutching the invitation, the reality of what happened sank in for the first time. Andrea was gone. She wouldn't be there to hold my hand on my wedding day. She wasn't going to be by my side when I said "I do" to the love of my life. She was dead. *Falleció*. I would never again be able to look into her dancing eyes or braid her thick brown hair. The realization hit me like a punch in the gut and I started wailing. The sound was that of a wounded animal; my soul was missing its mate.

I heard Ringo barking and I came to; Dennis was holding me. "Breathe," he said. "You have to breathe." I couldn't get a deep breath. There was no air. Andrea took it all with her. "You have to breathe!" Dennis said. "Breathe!" Finally, I was able to draw air into my lungs. I collapsed in Dennis's arms and cried until I fell into a dreamless sleep.

I was awakened the next morning by the sound of a bird's chirping. My head was throbbing. The green box with our wedding invitation was still open on the floor. I looked inside. Under the invitation were mementos from our time together at Envision Festival. The box was meant for me. I could tell. I piled everything back inside and stood to leave. That's when I saw it: there, in the corner of the room, was her yoga mat—the same gray mat she got for my retreat in Costa Rica in December. Andrea had been so excited to be there with me. She had been on retreats with me before but never joined an entire one. On the first day she grabbed me on the way to the yoga deck after breakfast. "Look what I got!" she cried. In her arms was the brand-new mat. "My own yoga mat! Aren't you proud of me?"

I rolled out the mat on the wood floor. It was a little dirty, like she'd just used it at the beach. I could see exactly where Andrea's hands had been in Child's Pose. I wasn't sure whether the angry scars from my surgery would allow me to do a single pose, but standing in her footprints, I started to move. Breathing deeply, I lifted my hands over my head. Soon I found my way into Downward-Facing Dog. As I aligned my body with my breath, I could feel the heaviness of my body. The weight of my heart, the pain; it felt unbearable. But somehow, I also knew it wasn't—because there I was, in it, feeling it all. Years of yoga practice had taught me just that: the art of breathing through discomfort. Of sitting with pain. Of breathing in to the tight corners of my body and making space wherever I need it. I realized, *this is it*. This is the point of all that practice. So that I could be here, right now, moving through this pain without having to escape.

Eventually I found myself in Savasana, resting my head where I knew Andrea had rested hers so many times before. Tears streaming down my face, I held my hands to my broken heart. Lying there on her mat, I knew what I had to do. I had to let myself feel. The only way out was through.

11

RELEASE

It was soon time to say good-bye to Costa Rica. As we were leaving Andrea's house, I remembered the beads I had left on the log when emptying the bag from the hospital. I walked out into the garden and picked one up. Looking at it I saw it was actually closer to pale blue than gray. Closing my fist around it, I could see Andrea dancing, her necklace swaying as she moved. "Good-bye," I whispered. "I'll be back soon." I put the bead in my pocket and left.

Dennis and I embarked on a yoga tour I had scheduled long ago, with workshops in Brazil, then back in Costa Rica, and finally Sweden. I felt an intense need to carry on, partly because I was terrified of what might happen if I wasn't in perpetual motion. I was spending more time on airplanes than I was with my feet on the ground, by my own choosing. Still, I was so tired I couldn't think straight. My skin broke out, my hair was oily, my hands were dry, my neck was stiff, and my stomach was tied in knots. But I was alive. My heart was beating. I was going through the most difficult time of my life, and I allowed myself to feel my feelings. When I needed to cry, I cried. When I wanted to laugh, I did. Most of the time I felt like a shaking leaf being blown around by the wind. But the wind was powerful and strong, and it was blowing with intention. I knew that letting go of control was how I would heal. I would let the uncertainty of the wind take me where I needed to go. One day at a time.

Neither Dennis nor I had ever been to Brazil before. I had committed to two workshops—one in Rio, the other in São Paulo. Both were sold out. I thought about canceling, but hundreds of people were coming. It would be a challenge to teach the classes. Not only was I in a fragile emotional state, they were handstand workshops and I hadn't even been able to do a proper vinyasa since my surgery, much less hold myself up in the air on my hands. But I wanted to go. I had to stay busy. Canceling didn't feel like an option.

We were late getting to the airport, which was unusual for us. Check-in had closed by the time we got to the counter and we had to plead for them to let us go through. "The plane is about to embark so if I were you I'd hurry up," the man at the check-in cautioned.

We had luggage, so Dennis told me to run ahead alone. "Hold the plane!" he called after me. "I'm right behind you!" I ran through security and to our gate. They were already paging us when Dennis called to tell me he wasn't allowed to pass through security because his US visa had expired. We had a layover in the United States and they wouldn't let him on without it.

There I was, about to make an eighteen-hour trip to a strange country with no Dennis and no luggage. I traveled alone all the time, but after Andrea died I felt too vulnerable to be on my own. I couldn't go to the grocery store by myself, let alone fly to Atlanta, change planes, and cross an entire continent.

I sank into my seat and tried to stay positive, but all I felt was panic. I started crying, and suddenly felt the walls of the plane shrinking. I couldn't breathe. What was I doing here? I was about to stand up to try to get off the plane when, suddenly, a sea of glittering light appeared all around me. It was everywhere—on the ceiling, the wall, the back of the seat in front of me. It stopped me right in my tracks, and for a moment, all I could see were the sparkles of light surrounding me. My panic subsided and I felt a warm, almost glowy feeling inside. I knew this light, I realized. It reminded me of the light that surrounded me when I jumped naked into the ocean after my surgery. Andrea. I felt her. It took me a while to realize that the light was bouncing off my engagement ring. But it was Andrea. I was sure of it. I said a silent prayer. *Thank you for showing me the light in the most difficult moments.* I had no idea if Dennis would make it to Brazil. All I knew was, in that moment, I was okay. I could take another breath. The plane took off and I opened my computer to read e-mails. Most were from people with messages about love and loss.

Reading them, I knew: I was not alone.

I landed in Rio, and Dennis, strangely, through some miracle, was already there. In his desperation, he managed to find a direct flight straight from Aruba to São Paulo that we didn't know existed and then he took a puddle jumper to Rio. We landed at the same time. It felt so serendipitous. Our hotel was on the ocean and we spent the first evening drinking caipirinhas and drunkenly making out in the middle of the street. I told him how I'd almost had a panic attack on the plane but that Andrea saved me. Holding his hand, walking down cobblestoned streets, I felt almost normal.

My class was the next morning. Some 250 people attended. It was my first big class since Andrea's accident. Dennis demonstrated the yoga poses for me since I still couldn't hold a handstand. I found myself thinking that sometimes it was hard being me. Everyone showed up expecting me to fix something for them—as if I held the keys to whatever they were looking for. Many were followers on Instagram and I was an inspiration for them. Some found their way to yoga through my posts. It had changed their lives and they credited me. But it wasn't me. I'm just like them, a regular person just trying to find her way.

Still, when I walked into the room, everyone stared. Some gasped, like they couldn't believe I was real. "Oh my God," said one young woman. "I can't believe this is happening! You're real! And Dennis! Hi! I'm sorry, this must be so weird for you. I feel like I know you so well, but you don't even know who I am." I smiled and gave her a hug. "No, it's not weird at all!" I said, even though she was right. It was weird. "It's so nice to meet you! Thank you so much for coming." I was being genuine; but I was also lying. It was strange, but it wasn't strange—I was used to doing it all the time: hug strangers and tell them it's not strange that they know my entire life, and now I've traveled across the world to teach them yoga, and they have spent money to be there, without a clue about whether I know what I'm talking about. It was a bit odd, but also awesome, the life I had managed to create for myself.

Walking into the room is always the hardest part, the anticipation, the excitement. At times I feel like I don't deserve it. Truth be told, I hate the attention. I just want to get to my mat so I can slip into the role of yoga teacher and get on with the class. I never truly relax until everyone is in their first pose, because then they're not thinking about me anymore. They're not thinking about Yoga Girl. They are focused on their breath and themselves. That's when I can be anonymous again. I dive into the part I love—the guiding, the breathing, the intention setting, the community, the movement. The poetry of speaking a language that surprises me every time I bring it forth. Sometimes I say things in class that I have no idea I ever knew.

This class, my first one since everything happened, is beautiful. I love everyone in the room. They are listening and so attentive. When it's time for Savasana everyone is sweaty, tired, present, emotional. Fully here. I crank up the music and "Spirit Bird" by Xavier Rudd fills the room. I walk around and give people adjustments, tiny groundings of the shoulders and gentle touches to the forehead, the neck. And suddenly, I see her. Andrea. The girl in front of me has a wooden earring in her ear. It's almost exactly the same as Andrea's—except I know it can't be, because hers was just a stick she found on the beach and shoved through her ear, and she was cremated with it. I smile and Andrea's presence fills the room. The next girl has tiny tattoos scattered across her forearms. They make no sense, their placement, it's like she's just sprinkled them across her arm. Andrea had similar tattoos. My heart beats a little faster. I move to the next girl, and the next, and the next. One has toes that are identical to Andrea's. Another, a single dread nestled in her messy hair. Like Andrea. Looking around, I notice that every person in this room has a piece of her. She is here. In all of us.

With the next person I adjust I feel like I'm having an out-of-body experience. I feel like I'm floating. I look down and there she is. I've been running in circles looking for her, but she's been there, in this girl, in me, all along. I start to cry. My tears drip onto the face of the girl beneath me. She grabs my hand and clutches it tightly. "It's okay," she says. "I lost my husband. I know. I am you, too." Now I'm sobbing and the whole room can hear me and Dennis is on the other side of the room, wondering if he needs to take over. I look at him and shake my head. No. I'm okay. There is no judgment here, just a room full of people breathing, feeling, living.

I wipe away my tears and stand up. I feel that fire within me. I go back to my mat at the front of the room and let it burn.

From Rio, we fly to São Paulo. It's very, very different. We're not on the beach anymore but in a giant city; it's dirty, but we meet nice people. They tell us it's not safe to leave our hotel at night. I've never traveled anywhere with fear and I'm not about to begin now.

Things didn't start off well. The woman who arranged for my class said she was having trouble with her bank accounts and didn't know how she would pay me. The event was over-sold and there was no greenroom or quiet area where I could go before class. Everywhere I went, people pulled at me and insisted on taking selfies. The excitement felt almost aggressive, but I had to smile and look serene because that's what people expected of Yoga Girl. I just wanted to take a breath and pre-pare for class, but there wasn't a private space, and time was short.

Things went from bad to worse. When it was time to start, the hosts gave me a headset but the mic didn't work. I was standing in front of five hundred people who couldn't hear me. I tried to joke my way through it, but no one laughed. Finally, someone gave me a handheld mic, which meant I couldn't use my hands while I taught; I couldn't reach my hands up, or demonstrate a pose, or place my hands on my heart, or adjust the students. I pride myself on being able to create an intimate space even in classes of that size. If people don't cry during my classes, if they aren't able to arrive at a place inside of them-selves where they feel so much it overflows, I feel as though I've failed. How would I ever make this an intimate, genuine experience? I had no idea. But the show had to go on.

I walked around, feeling like a clown. I said the right words, and we did what we were supposed to do, but something was so totally off. Several people had their phones on their mats and when I walked by, they took photos of me, right in the middle of their practice. I had never experienced anything like it. I felt violated.

On the verge of tears, all I could think was that I wanted to go home. Normally, after we bow our heads at the end of a session, people take a moment to breathe, to gather themselves. Sometimes we follow up with a brief Q&A, and after that, I hug people and we take photos. But for this class, I barely got to open my eyes after I'd said *namaste* before people had left their mats and were shoving their phones in my face.

I had nowhere to go—no way to escape. Before I knew it, throngs of people surrounded me. A sort of hysteria was building. Someone grabbed the side of my head with such force I thought I heard the vertebrae in my neck pop—and not in a good way. Hundreds of people were pressing up against me like an angry mob, screaming for photographs. At one point, I was dragged down and feared I would be trampled. When I surfaced again, I caught Dennis's eye across the room. He looked panicked. "Do something!" he screamed at the promoter. "Get her out of there!" *I'm not a human being anymore*, I thought. I'm some Internet celebrity they need a photograph with to prove to their friends they were here. There is no yoga happening in this room. "You have to let me out of here," I cried.

Finally, thankfully, the crowd dispersed enough for Dennis to get to me. He picked me up and fished me out of the crowd. "This is over. Move!" he shouted, putting me down on the stairs. A girl held up her phone. "But I didn't get a photo yet!" she said angrily. Hearing the disappointment in her voice made me feel awful.

I hurried upstairs to the bathroom, sat on a toilet, and wrapped my arms around my legs. I had just been pushed down, had my head jacked and my hair pulled, but I felt an obligation to go back and give more of myself. A few minutes later, the crowd was still there. People were still aiming their phones. "You don't have to do this," Dennis said. "You don't owe these people anything. Let's just go."

I walked back down the stairs and stepped into the crowd.

From Brazil, we flew back to Costa Rica for another retreat. When my last class ended in Dominical, I had convinced Dennis to join Cado on a surfing trip they'd planned months earlier. He hadn't had a moment to himself since Andrea died, and I knew he needed his own time to process, too. It couldn't have been easy, holding our little family together. Ringo and I took a shuttle bus up to San José to spend more time with Andrea's family. We were halfway there when Luigi called. "I'm picking you up at the station," he said.

I'd been angry with Luigi since Andrea's accident. The three of us had been inseparable and now he was completely distant. Every time I'd seen him since Andrea died he had acted strange, almost cold. He kept asking about me and how I was coping but refused to talk about himself. Actually, he didn't even want to mention Andrea's name. I had thought I'd find relief with Luigi, knowing he was one of the only people who knew Andrea the way I did, but instead I felt like he was someone I didn't know. It was like our relationship had died with Andrea. The last time he and I had been together I accused him of being uncaring and he'd stalked away.

I was surprised when he called, and not sure how I would feel when I saw him. He was waiting when the bus arrived in

San José. I had barely gotten myself and Ringo settled in the car when he started talking. As he spoke, tears spilled down his cheeks. I'd never seen him cry before, not once. "I'm sorry," he said. "When they told me she didn't make it, the first thing I thought of was you. I knew you wouldn't be okay, no way, never. Me? I can shut down, soldier on, continue. You? I knew it would kill you. I couldn't cry with you because I knew it would break me and you would feel like you had to pick up the pieces. I didn't want that. So I had to be cold. And strong. So I wouldn't fall apart. But I realize now that I made everything worse."

So many things ran through my mind as he spoke. I understood now that caring for me was a coping mechanism for him. If he just focused on me, helped me, he wouldn't have to process the fact that his best friend died, too. It was messed up, but I understood. "I just wanted you to be there," I said. "I just can't believe this happened. Us. Our family. Our family time. How are we going to live now?" Tears fell into my lap as I spoke. He wrapped his arm around me. "I don't know," he said. "I miss her so much. She was the most alive person I've ever known. I still can't believe it's real. And a part of me wants to turn around and run away, because being with you is being with her and it hurts. It's hard to be here, with you, because it reminds me that she is not here anymore. And it's so painful."

I was staying at Andrea's house that night. I wanted to spend time there before her family closed it up for good. Luigi and I stayed in the car talking until it got dark and cold. I invited him inside and we cooked dinner, but I was too emotionally drained to even get a fork to my mouth.

I walked upstairs to Andrea's room. It was just as I'd left

it a few weeks earlier. I opened her closet and the smell of her almost knocked me off my feet. I drank it in. It was like she was right here. I leaned into the closet and wrapped my arms around her dresses. I wanted to wear all of them. I had an overwhelming urge to put every item on the bed and sleep on them. Andrea's mom had told me to take everything that meant anything to me, but I decided to gather only a few things. I already had her Guatemalan leather pouch—it had been hanging on my hip since the last time I was at the house. And her yoga mat and wooden mala beads. Going through her closet, a few things popped out: The long pink and yellow scarf with the little bells on the ends. She wore it at Envision and we used it as a towel to lie on at the beach after swimming naked one afternoon. I took it from the closet and wrapped it around my neck. The black dress, the one I bought her for her birthday; I have an identical one. The green top she wore all the time. The short skirt she bartered for at the festival. The pajama pants with little reindeer I always borrowed. Once I'd started, I couldn't stop. I pulled out a purple sweater I'd never seen her wear. A white top that was braided like a leaf in the back. An orange dress. Jeans. She never wore jeans. I thought if I just found the right thing, the thing that had been closest to her, maybe she'd come alive again if I wore it.

After a while I couldn't even see what was on the hangers I was pulling down because I was crying too hard. A wail came out of me that was so loud I surprised myself. I dropped down on the floor, surrounded by her things, and something that was already broken inside of me broke again. Andrea felt so close but so far away. Suddenly, Luigi was by my side. He hugged me and let me cry. When I ran out of tears I fell asleep right there as I was, lying in the pile of Andrea's clothes, my arms wrapped around dresses she would never wear again. When I awakened I was on the floor, freezing. It was three in the morning, three hours until my flight was scheduled to leave. Luigi and I decided to go outside and wait. I went out on the balcony and lay in the hammock. Luigi followed me. "Scooch," he said, and laid down. I had no energy left to cry. My body felt like it weighed a thousand pounds. I was numb. I rested my head on Luigi's shoulder, about to ask him what we were going to do now, how we would ever live again, because life without her was unthinkable, when suddenly, his lips met mine. I was so stunned I didn't know what was happening. For a second, I kissed him back. It wasn't a kiss of passion, nor attraction or romance. It was a kiss of the most intense sadness I had ever experienced. We were two people moving through grief, and for a second, the intimacy became so intense and vulnerable that our lips just merged. It was brief. I came to my senses and pulled away. None of it made sense. I had a fiancé whom I was very much in love with. "What are we doing?" I asked. "This is not us." "I don't know," he said, tears in his eyes. "I'm sorry."

Standing, I walked to the other side of the balcony. Looking out at the jungle, I heard Andrea's voice in my head: *Grief is not an excuse to act like an asshole!* Of course she was right. I needed to get my shit together. I heard Luigi behind me. "Andrea would hate this," Luigi said. "She would say, grief isn't an excuse to act like assholes." I smiled. "I was just thinking the same thing," I said. He gave me a sad smile. "Alright. Back to reality. Let's pack up."

We put all of Andrea's things back in the closet. In the end, I took only a few things: The pajama pants. The green top. The black dress. The sun was about to rise. It was time to go. We were headed downstairs when something caught my eye. The faux fur. The hairs stood up on the back of my neck. Our all-time favorite vest. I ran over and reached up to grab it. It was a huge faux fur vest with a giant hood that we always wore out dancing—my favorite was wearing almost nothing else, just a bikini or short-shorts with the vest. And boots. We had so much fun dressing up with it. I wrapped my arms around the vest and inhaled. It smelled like us. I put it on and turned to look at Luigi. Tears were running down his face. "You look so much like her," he said. "I see her. In you. All the time."

I knew exactly what he meant. I felt like her, too.

Luigi dropped me at the airport. "I hope I didn't fuck anything up," he said. I saw worry in his eyes. Had we ruined something? I answered, "You didn't. Everything is already fucked up. I'll see you soon."

I was at customs with Ringo when we were pulled aside. "Papers, please," the officer said.

I handed them Ringo's health certificate, passport, and vaccination book. After a while they returned. "We need the SENASA form signed by the Costa Rican veterinarian." I didn't know what they were talking about. I took Ringo everywhere with me and never had a problem. He'd been to Costa Rica more times than I could count. It was five thirty in the morning and my flight was leaving in forty minutes. I was wearing a giant fur vest, yoga pants, and woven boots. My eyes were red from crying, my face was puffy from lack of sleep. The security man looked at me with sympathy. Turns out, Costa Rica had a new law that required pets to get checked out by a local vet ten days prior to traveling. "I'm so sorry, miss, but I can't let you pass," he said. "You will have to go get your papers signed and book a new flight ten days from today. There is no way you'll be getting on a plane today. Not unless you want to leave the dog behind."

His words triggered in me a full-blown meltdown. Having gone through so much pain and such an emotional roller coaster for so many weeks—I just didn't give a shit about what people thought anymore. I started bawling. All-out hysterical bawling. The security guy didn't know what to do. "Miss, please . . . I didn't mean to make you upset." I barely heard him. "It's just ten days," he said. "I know it seems like a lot, but I really can't let you through."

I kept crying. After a while the security officer left and came back with another officer. I sat on the floor, clutching Ringo. After a while the crying stopped, but I didn't. I was faking crying noises. I wanted people to think I was a little crazy. *Who gives a flying fuck anyway?* I thought. People were walking past, staring at me. I kicked off my boots and let out a grunt. It was, admittedly, a little pathetic. I'd become one of those people who have public meltdowns! I was a complete mess. The thought of not going home, of having yet another obstacle in my way was the proverbial straw that broke the camel's back. I'd been doing a pretty good job keeping myself together up until then. For all the crying I'd done in public, this took the cake. I leaned back and closed my eyes. I'd been on the floor long enough that I'd probably missed my flight. I decided to just stay there. *What are they going to do to me?* I thought. *Force me out of the airport? There is nothing anyone can do that will hurt more than I already do.*

When I opened my eyes again the security guy was standing there. He looked over his shoulder to make sure no one was watching and handed me Ringo's papers. "Go," he said. I pouted. "I'm not going anywhere," I said. "I have no place to go and you can't force me to leave." I looked up at him. "I thought you had a flight to catch," he said. I couldn't believe it. "You're . . . letting me go?" "Yes," he said. "Go now. Before I change my mind." I jumped up and gathered my things: my fur, my boots, my carry-on, my leather pouch, my Italian greyhound. I looked like a one-woman traveling circus. "Thank you!" I said. He put his hand on my shoulder. "Whatever it is, it's going to get better," he said, then turned and walked away. I ran to my gate. The plane was waiting. They were calling my name.

I was home in Aruba for only a couple of days before we were off again, this time for the last leg of the tour in my homeland. Besides my business obligations, Dennis and I had a wedding to prepare for! It was the last time we'd be in Sweden before we returned that summer for our ceremony. We still had to arrange for flowers, and cake, and music. More than two hundred people were on our guest list and people would be flying in from twelve different countries. I felt good about being busy, but I was hardly myself. We went to bakeries to choose the cake, but everything felt generic and boring. I got so frustrated during one of the tastings that I snapped at the server. "This is not what you promised us!" I said. "We were supposed to try the varieties promised in our confirmation e-mail. This is *not* it!" As I spoke, my eyes burned with tears. "Is there a reason you are serving us what we didn't order?" I was lashing out and I couldn't stop myself. I knew I was behaving badly and I didn't care. "Maybe we should take our business to a place that actually cares about its customers!" I said. Dennis excused us and we went outside. "*What* is going on? Why are you so angry at that waitress?" he asked. "It's not a big deal! We'll find a good cake. You have to stop acting like this." I started to cry. "It's too much," I said. "I don't know how to do this." I made myself go back in and apologize. I felt like I'd completely lost the ability to manage social situations. I didn't know how to deal with people. I didn't know how to deal with myself.

That evening, Dennis was quiet. "Do you want to postpone the wedding?" he asked with tears in his eyes. I was stunned. "Maybe you are right. Maybe this is too much," he said. "This is supposed to be a happy time. It's supposed to be the happiest time of our lives." I could see the pain in his eyes as he spoke. Postponing the wedding was not what I wanted. "No. No!" I cried. "Absolutely not. I'm sorry. I wish we didn't have to go through this. I wish it wasn't this hard." He pulled me close. "Thank God you didn't say you wanted to postpone the wedding," he said. "That would have killed me." It felt unfair. Regular people get to plan their weddings and feel excited about what's ahead. Why did the happiest moment of my life have to be combined with the saddest?

We finally made it back to Aruba and I tried to make my way to some kind of normalcy. I'd roll out my mat in the mornings to try and find my way back to the practice. Sometimes, moving my body and breathing deeply helped. Sometimes, sitting on my yoga mat made me want to scream. I continued to share my sadness with my followers. Sometimes it was the only thing that could give me any relief. People sent me things. Letters. Little gifts. Paintings. Pieces of jewelry. Gemstones. For Yoga Girl. I wrote on Instagram two or three times every day, but I wasn't objectively connected to the fact that a million people were reading my thoughts every day. For me, it was just a process and it had become part of my healing. I'd feel a wave of grief coming, and if it got so bad I didn't know what to do with myself, instead of panicking I would reach for my phone and type while the tears flowed. Reading people's comments helped me to remember what I already knew: We all feel the same things. Just not always at the same time. We all, at one point in our lives, go through hell and back. We're all human. I was not alone.

Not everyone was patient with me, however. Some in my social media community had grown tired of my grief. One woman urged me to return to posting inspiring things, the way I had done before tragedy struck, "because if it was you who died in that car crash, and not your best friend, what kind of post would you want to leave as your last?" I'd lost more than a hundred thousand followers in the weeks since Andrea's death. I was sorry to lose so many virtual friends, but not enough to change my ways. *I'm just a regular person;*

just like anyone else, I told myself. I have good days and bad days and I tried to be real and honest with my ups and downs. My goal is to inspire, but if I'm not real, what's the point? If I lost some followers along the way, it would have to be okay. It meant the real people stayed. Moving through this kind of pain brought with it an intense urge to be myself—I didn't have time to fake it for anyone. I didn't want to pretend. I knew now, life is short. I wasn't going to waste it bending over backward trying to please people. I realized just how much time I had spent in my life worried about whether people liked me; if I was doing the right thing; if I was good enough. I'd worry about not being thin enough, successful enough, special enough for other people to like me. But what about me? Did I like me? After all, my relationship with myself was the most important one and I could feel it in my bones: every time I tried to please someone else at my own expense, I was betraying myself. I was done posting things to social media because I hoped people would respond well to it or feel inspired by it. I only wanted to share whatever was authentic to my heart, every day. People could take it or leave it.

I saw the same change take place in my relationships; shallow friendships that I'd stayed in out of habit or because of mutual history ("we've been friends for so long!") began to fall away. It wasn't that those friends had changed. I had. I couldn't partake in shallow conversation anymore. I only wanted to surround myself with people who were able to sit with the real me—with all of me. Not just my happiness and my gratitude and my joy, but also my sadness and confusion and despair.

Real friends know how to love all of you. And I knew in my core that cultivating those relationships meant I had to begin with me. I had to love all of me. Every time I chose myself, every time I let myself be who I was, unapologetically . . . I moved a little bit closer to that place of self-love.

12

BELIEVE

Dennis and I flew to Sweden again in early June to get ready for the wedding later that month. We took Ringo with us and, for the first time, Pepper, too. Pepper had grown into a big dog—a black, Labrador-type giant, and he'd never been on a plane before. Getting married without him was never an option. We stayed at a hotel in downtown Stockholm, with all our suitcases and two dogs, because we wanted our own space, rather than to crowd into my mom's tiny apartment, or go farther out into the countryside with my dad. As soon as we landed I got a tattoo: the phases of the moon lined up across my forearm. The moon was a part of my connection to Andrea. Her Instagram account was @ahlaluna, her initials followed by the words "the moon" in Spanish, but I used to make fun of her and exclaim "ah, la luna," throwing my arm across my forehead with flair. It always made her giggle. She was a sister of the moon and took part in big women's gatherings every year, and she was the one to teach me how as women, our menstrual cycles connect with the moon. The tattoo not only reminded me that just like the moon, life waxes and wanes in cycles—what comes, must go, and come again—but also, every night the moon rises, giving me an opportunity to talk to her.

With the wedding two weeks away, my to-do list was endless: seating charts to make, transportation to be booked and hotel rooms reserved, little gift bags to pack, decorations to buy. Last-minute changes were piling up, too, complicating our already hectic schedule: people who said they wouldn't be able to make it had suddenly changed their plans, and the castle where the celebration was taking place didn't have enough space, or staff, or plates and silverware, to accommodate everyone. The clock was ticking and I still didn't have a wedding dress. Not "the dress." I had just sort of surrendered to the idea that I'd wear a dress I brought with me. It was pretty enough, but I just wasn't feeling it. With so much on my mind, at least I didn't have to think as much about how sad I was, which was a nice reprieve.

The weekend before the wedding was midsummer, a big celebration in Sweden. I took the dogs and my friend Amelie out to my friend's island in the archipelago for the weekend. Amelie was a new friend. She'd come to my retreat in Costa Rica a few months earlier, when Andrea was there, and we'd stayed in touch. Over the last few weeks, she had made herself indispensable with wedding planning and she'd become a shoulder for me to lean on.

The island celebration was nice, but it felt odd that no one mentioned Andrea. Everyone knew my best friend had died, but enough time had passed that people just didn't think to ask anymore. Which was strange, because in my world, no time had passed at all. Everyone was drinking and talking about superficial things that, in the big scheme of life, didn't matter—but they hadn't just lost someone, so they weren't thinking that none of it mattered. To me, the conversations and the wine and the laughter all echoed with shallow nothing.

At one point, I sat on the dock alone and cried. Unbeknownst to me, my friend Daniella snapped a photo of me facing away from the crowd, thinking I was sitting on the dock in meditation. In the picture, a giant orb sits beneath my shoulders, right at the back of my heart. Since Andrea died, those little orbs kept showing up in my photos. People said it was just an iPhone thing but I knew better. It was the same light that glittered across the ocean as the sun set. The same light I saw on the windows, walls, and ceiling of the airplane. It was the air I'd forgotten I knew how to breathe. It was Andrea.

When we got back to Stockholm, I decided to get another tattoo. It was a spontaneous one (the moon phases I had long envisioned inked on my arm). Dennis and I were walking down Södermalm. It was sunny and our friends had begun to arrive from other countries. It was just such a good day. The chorus I'd had in the back of my mind for the last three months came to me as we were walking, lyrics from the song "Black as Night." "I believe in the good things coming, coming, coming, coming." Just as it came into my mind, I looked up and saw a sign for tattoos. "Let's go in," I said. Twenty minutes later, I was sitting in the chair. I asked the artist if I could play the song while he inked me. "My friend died," I said. "This was our song." The tattoo artist looked at me. "Of course," he said.

"Play it loud, man." And I did. I wanted to feel her presence. I wanted to believe in the good things coming. I turned up the music as he put the needle to my skin. I left with the words "I believe in the good things coming" wrapped around my left forearm, right below the crease of my elbow.

Suddenly it was two days and counting. Dennis still needed a haircut; I needed a manicure; we were missing hotel rooms for five guests; people were asking for directions; the seating chart needed to be updated yet again to accommodate last-minute attendees; Dennis didn't have a tie; I didn't have the right underwear.

On the way to get my nails done, I envisioned myself walking down the aisle in the castle gardens, Dennis waiting for me by the water. I tried to see myself in the dress I had hanging in the closet. It wasn't quite right, but I decided I would just have to learn to love it. At the same time I was thinking about the dress, my phone rang. The call was from Amelie. "Something amazing just happened!" she yelled excitedly when I picked up. "Ida Sjöstedt is opening her bridal studio for you and is offering you a dress!" "*What?*" I asked. It couldn't be true. Ida Sjöstedt is one of the most renowned couture designers in Sweden—her dresses are a literal bohemian dream. But they go for ten thousand dollars easily. "They said to come to the studio and if you find the one you love, you can have it," Amelie said. I couldn't believe what I was hearing. "She follows you on Instagram," Amelie continued breathlessly. "She's been reading your story." It turned out that Amelie had a connection to the designer's studio. "I felt called to check in, so I did and they had seen a post from you that you were getting married.

They said we should come right over. Isn't that so strange?" I smiled. "Let's go!" I said.

I moved my nail appointment and met Amelie at the bridal studio. I found "the dress" immediately. Two pieces. A strapless hand-stitched lace top that clung to my waist over a wide and flowy tulle skirt. I felt like a fairy princess in it. It was the most beautiful dress I had ever seen. And it was offered to me as a gift. I took the dress back to the hotel room and gave myself a moment to breathe. There was so much energy buzzing inside me; I didn't know how to wind down. The dress felt like a miracle. Actually, there had been miracles all around. *I should be writing all of this down*, I thought to myself. *To make sure I won't forget.* I lay on the bed and closed my eyes. I was so tired from the emotional roller coaster of the last few months, but also so happy about what was ahead.

I had begun to nod off when I was startled by the sound of my phone. Olivia, my maid of honor, was calling. "Hey, do you have your something blue yet?" she asked. "If not we've got to find something today." I had something borrowed—a golden crown for my hair. My dress was something new. My ring, something old. It belonged to my grandmother. But I didn't have something blue. Olivia and I made plans to meet up to find that missing something. I hung up the phone, sat up, and reached for Andrea's pouch on the way out the door. When I did, something fell out and rolled under the bed. I crawled after it, expecting to see a coin. What I discovered was much more precious. There, underneath the bed, was a small blue-gray bead. It took me a moment to recognize it. It was that tiny bead from Andrea's necklace, the one she wore on the morning of the crash. The bead I took with me from the log in the garden outside her house, from her torn necklace. The bead from the necklace I pulled out of a bag marked "Medical Waste." The hairs on my arms stood up. I didn't know I had it. I thought it was safe on my altar at home in Aruba. Apparently it had been in the pouch, hanging on my hip, all along. My something blue. I called Olivia. "You're not going to believe this," I said.

On Friday, we drove to the castle. The pre-wedding fes-tivities were starting. Lejondal Castle is located just north of Stockholm and we found it on a whim. I know it sounds very fairy tale–like, getting married in a castle, but Sweden is a mon-archy with a proper king and queen, and castles are all over the country. Most have been converted to spas and hotels or event halls, like the one where we were about to be married. It was nestled right on a lake, surrounded by forest and greenery. The castle gardens are beautiful and we were planning to have the ceremony outside. There would be a white-sand aisle and I'd planned to be barefoot.

I had butterflies in my stomach when we checked in. The place was alive with preparation. Our room overlooked the water. We dropped our bags and went for a walk with the dogs—they were overjoyed to have left the city for the country. Pepper was such a good dog. He never needed to be on a leash, and Ringo never left his side.

That evening we gathered with our guests in the court-yard for a rustic summer barbecue; we drank strawberry-lime caipirinhas out of mason jars and enjoyed a buffet of whole-roasted corn, veggie skewers, portobello mushrooms, and fresh local fish. The venue was decorated beautifully. String lights flickered all around the gardens. Two hundred people had come to celebrate our love. Friends from Aruba, Costa Rica, Holland, the United States, Canada, the UK, Spain, Norway, South Africa, India . . . It was a perfect evening—everything I ever could have imagined. The plan was to wrap up the party early so everyone could get to bed at a decent hour and be ready for the big wedding. We ended up dancing until three in the morning—to this day, the party on the eve before our wedding is the best party we've ever been to.

The next morning I woke up early but didn't feel tired. I walked out on the balcony and looked at the lake. It was still, not a ripple across the surface. I smiled, thinking of the festivities that had continued late into the night—and it was just the beginning! I felt calm.

We finished breakfast just in time for morning yoga. With so many of our friends being yoga instructors, we planned for a yoga session every day. Mats were laid out across the lawn and twenty or so of our guests joined in. I always set an intention at the start of my practice. Usually it's something related to my body, or to flow, to let something go, to feel strong, to feel calm. On this day, it was very simple. Love. Just love. We flowed and stretched and moved and breathed and when we were done and lying in Savasana, my heart was pounding so hard it felt like it might shoot out of my chest. Dennis reached for my hand. I squeezed it tightly. The love I felt for him . . . I couldn't find the words for it. It was bigger than anything I'd ever experienced before. Somehow, even with everything we'd been through over the past months, I was overcome with a feeling of purpose. We were here for a reason. This was the right place. The right time. Him and I. Forever. Opening my eyes, I saw the sky above me. Blades of grass tickled my fingers. The earth felt like it was vibrating. I was so, so happy. I realized; it is possible to move through grief, and still feel joy. To hold space for sadness and gratitude at the same time. To miss someone and still be happy for the ones that are near. I was feeling it all.

When Dennis headed off with his groomsmen to get ready, I took my girls to my room. The bridesmaids' dresses were dusty blue, just what Andrea wanted. All the dresses were on hangers, just steamed. Everyone took their dresses, one by one, and for a moment we stood there, holding our dresses, looking at the rack. One dress was left. Andrea's dress. I closed my eyes and imagined her walking in at any moment. When I opened them again, everyone was crying. We hugged, and looking at my bridesmaids, I realized I'd been so focused on the one I was missing that I hadn't paid enough attention to the ones still here. "I love you so much," I said. "Thank you for being here." I was grateful for so much. I was hours away from marrying the love of my life. My friends were here, our families, all our loved ones. Yes, I had lost one of my best friends. But I still had so much.

The hour leading up to the ceremony was fraught with typical wedding-day disasters. The minister was on time, but the wedding certificate was missing; the flower arrangements were not what we ordered; Dennis misplaced his cuff links; the arch was knocked over by the wind; and, finally, it started to rain. I felt my eyes starting to tear up when someone came bearing gifts. Luigi. "Gifts from San José," he said, hugging me tightly. The box was from Andrea's family. Inside was a letter signed by everyone in her family, sharing their love for Dennis and me, and a framed photo of Andrea—the one that was on the altar in the house when I first arrived there after her funeral. In it, Andrea has a scarf wrapped over her head and she is looking out into the distance. It's the most beautiful, serene picture. Also tucked inside the box was a copy of the book she had been reading before she died—meditations in Spanish about how to open your heart through merging with the present moment. Lastly, the most beautiful of gifts: bracelets that Andrea's cousin made using Andrea's own thread, the same thread she had wrapped in her hair. Three bracelets were for me and one was for Dennis. I slipped mine on my wrists and sent the one to Dennis in his room. We took the framed photo of Andrea and set up a little altar in the castle where we hung her dress and lit a candle. That way, everyone attending the wedding could take a moment throughout the celebration to sit with her.

In the moments before I walked down the aisle, I posted a photo of the little pale blue bead. Magically, someone had offered to turn it into a necklace just a few days earlier and now it was hanging around my neck. My something blue.

As we were about to leave the room, everyone turned quiet. "Group hug!" someone said. And then we were outside. It had stopped raining.

I'm barefoot walking through the grass, and when I turn the corner I see everyone seated for the ceremony. The sand is white, the arch is standing, and Dennis is waiting. He has tears in his eyes. I am so happy. My dad walks me down the aisle and squeezes my hand tight. When it's time for him to go sit down he forgets and stands there with us for the whole ceremony. Dennis is so handsome. For a moment, the sun comes out. I say "I do" with no hesitation.

It's the happiest day of my life.

13
___

ACCEPT

My grandmother is dying. She has been for a long time, but right now, we can all sense that the end is near. Death is on my doorstep once again.

When Mormor was younger, she was tall and lean and always wore skirts. She was alone, but I don't know if she was lonely. She divorced my grandfather when my mom was only three, and he died before I was born. She never remarried and I don't remember her ever having a partner or a boyfriend when I was growing up. For the longest time she lived alone in a great apartment in the center of Stockholm. One day she decided it was time for her to go to a retirement community—she didn't want to be alone anymore. We were all surprised because she managed so well and she was still young in our eyes. My mom and her sisters helped her get a place at a senior living facility outside of Uppsala. It was the kind where you have your own apartment and your own life but there are nurses on staff and a communal area where you can take your meals with your neighbors if you want—assisted living.

Mormor's next-door neighbor was a gentleman in his late seventies. His name was Sten. Within a week of her moving in, she called my mom to tell her that she and Sten had "struck up a friendship." They had found love. Mormor told me it was the first time she had ever been in love in her entire life and it happened when she was seventy-five years old. And for the last years of her life, she was happy.

She had been sick for some time; one thing after another, but she "hung in there," as she said. After breaking her hip she wasn't able to walk anymore and she'd been in a wheelchair for the last two years. More recently, she'd gotten an infection that wouldn't go away and she never really recovered. Still, right before we left Aruba for Sweden for the wedding, I was shocked when my mom called to say Mormor was moved to a hospice. "A hospice?" I cried. "But that's where people die!"

When Dennis and I first landed in Sweden for the wedding, we drove straight there from the airport. When I saw Mormor, my heart dropped. The last time I'd seen her was my previous visit to Sweden and, sure, she was in a wheelchair, but she was herself. She looked good, and she was laughing and making jokes and drank her tea with lots of sugar the way she always had. Now, lying in the big hospice bed, she looked tiny. She must have lost half of her body weight. I barely recognized her. When she saw me her face lit up. "You're here!" she said. "Rakis. Min älskling." *Rakis* was her nickname for me when I was little. "I'm here," I said, taking her hand. "I'm so happy you are marrying Dennis," she said. "I have a dress all ready that I'm going to wear. It's orange. I don't know where it is. Can you help me find it?" My eyes welled up. The chances of her making it to the wedding were slim. "I'll help you find it," I said. She saw Dennis and tried to sit up. "Dennis!" she cried. "Come give me a hug!" Everyone in my family loves Dennis. My grandma especially did. "It's so nice to see you," she said in English. "You both take care of each other. Promise me that."

Leaning back, she closed her eyes. "I have to find my orange dress," she said, drifting off. I put my head next to hers on her pillow. She opened her eyes briefly. "Promise you will come back," she said.

"I promise."

By the time of the wedding, Mormor hadn't spoken or opened her eyes for days. We decided not to postpone our honeymoon. It felt okay to go and I knew she would hate it if we didn't.

Before our flight, we return to the hospice to see her. She looks even smaller than the last time. All of my aunts are there, and my mom. They say any day now, and I believe it. We wheel her bed out into the garden and my aunt Stina starts tweezing little hairs from my grandmother's chin. It makes me smile. We all have them, these little black hairs that grow from our chins. It's the family curse—all the women are blessed with having to tweeze long man-hairs from our faces by the ripe old age of fourteen. My grandmother used to ask us to pluck them because she couldn't see them. She wouldn't want black hairs on her face when she is dying.

Eventually everyone else leaves and it's just us. I wonder if Mormor's feet are cold so I wrap my hands around her feet to warm them up. Her feet are big, two sizes bigger than mine. I close my eyes and breathe and through her feet I feel her. She is breathing and alive, but she is in transition. I wrap a blanket around her legs and tuck her in. I take her hand in mine and for a long time, we sit there. I tell her about the wedding and how beautiful it was. I say she would have loved the cake, and that we wish she could have been there, and that her orange dress would have looked so beautiful next to mine. I tell her about the speeches, and the stars above the castle, and the ceremony, and that it started to rain and then it didn't. I tell her everything and that I'm happy but I'm sad and a little scared. I tell her that I love her and that I am so grateful to have her in my life.

Her breathing is so slow. I try to sync mine up with hers and, after a while, I feel like I'm doing my pranayama, my breathing exercises from yoga. I find the kumbhaka, the pause between each breath. I am intensely present with her breath and mine. She is dying, but she is going somewhere. I feel that. I squeeze her hand and kiss her forehead. This is our good-bye.

That night Dennis and I left to spend five weeks abroad. We hadn't planned much. A few days before, we pulled up a world map and decided on Greece. Dennis had never been and I longed for the Mediterranean Sea. I used to go to Greece as a child, my mom and my little brother and I. We'd go island hopping and sleep on big boats under the stars with nothing but our backpacks. As a teenager I'd been back many times—I always felt a special pull toward Greece. I wanted to drink retsina by the sea. We decided on Santorini and two days before we were set to depart, I randomly e-mailed hotels. We booked five nights at a place that looked beautiful online, choosing to not make any further plans than that and just see where the journey takes us. We left Pepper and Ringo at my dad's place. He lives in the middle of the forest by a lake and there'd be plenty of space for them to roam and squirrels to chase.

We landed in Santorini in the middle of the night. Even at two in the morning, the airport was buzzing. Santorini is a big tourist destination, but we were headed to a hotel at the south end of the island, where it was quiet. When I looked back at the past year, I realized I hadn't been still for even a second. I traveled and saw amazing places, but I kept going going going. This honeymoon was the first time I was off— not working, not planning for the wedding, not teaching—in more than three years. I needed peace. We pulled into the hotel and it was pitch-black outside—I couldn't see a thing. But I could hear the ocean, and when we were shown our room I felt like I was in a dream. The walls were brick, the bed was crisp and white, and there was a big Jacuzzi in the middle of the room made of something that looked like cobblestone. Everything was rustic but luxurious with soft, warm lighting. Dennis and I collapsed on the bed. We were tired but in love, and before I drifted off to sleep I thought to myself, *Forever doesn't scare me anymore.*

I woke up with the sunrise. Dennis was still sleeping, so I slipped into a dress and quietly stepped outside. I opened the door to the patio and discovered that we were perched on a cliff that dropped hundreds of feet into the ocean. I knew we were by the sea, but I had no idea I would be waking up to this. Vast, sapphire-blue ocean for as far as the eye could see. The sun was rising on the horizon. The wind was strong. I stepped up on the ledge and looked down. Waves crashed on the pebbled beach far, far below. The sun hit my face and for a moment, everything was quiet. I felt the breath in my lungs, and the slow pace of each inhale and exhale. My heart felt full. Suddenly, I felt the space between my grandmother's breaths, the way I had when I last sat by her bedside. I closed my eyes and somehow . . . I knew. There was no breath left in her lungs anymore. There was only space now. Mormor was gone. It was July sixth. Her birthday.

I stood there for a long, long time. Not feeling over-whelmed with sadness but crying with knowing. Dennis came outside, holding my phone. "Dushi . . ." he said. "Sweetheart" or "sweetie" in Papiamento, his native language. The look on his face was pained and there was a deep furrow between his brows. "I know," I said. "It's okay. I know." He hugged me. He is so tall. My husband. His arms are so big. I always feel tiny in his arms. I wiped the tears from my face.

When I heard my mother's voice I could hear her pain. She doesn't do well with tragedy, with death. She cried, but sounded calm. I asked if I should come home, holding my breath, hop-ing she would say not to, because if she didn't, I wouldn't be able to stay where I was. It was part of our relationship, my wanting to fix her, to save her. It was the part that weighed me down. "No," she said. "Stay in Greece." I sighed with relief.

It was our honeymoon and my grandmother had passed away and somehow, I was okay. I had to remind myself that life never gives you anything you cannot handle and that all I could do was trust in both endings and beginnings. In the end isn't that what we are all here to do? To love and to say good-bye and to love again. To love and let go, love and let go, love and let go . . . It's the single most important thing we can learn in this lifetime.

14

PRAY

Greece, Italy, Spain, Morocco, France. It had been one hell of a honeymoon. Five weeks abroad. We returned to Stockholm, ready to pick up the dogs and go home. Pepper and Ringo were overjoyed to see us. Pep howled with happiness when he saw our car pull in, and then ran in circles around us on the lawn. Ringo crawled up under my sweater. I love my babies so much.

After dinner with my dad and some of our friends, Dennis and I started packing to go home. I decided to leave our wedding gifts and my wedding dress behind until next time, but still, after hours of careful packing, we had five suitcases. I was really, really looking forward to going home.

We hugged the family good-bye and got on the plane. Pepper lay quietly by my feet. All I could think about was what a good dog he was. Halfway through the flight, the flight attendant asked, "Is he sick?" "No, no," I said. "He's just a really good boy." She scratched his ear and Pepper licked her hand. "He's just so quiet. I've never seen a dog so calm!" An hour or two later she returned to ask if he wanted some water. "No, thank you," I said. "I give him some every other hour or so." She looked concerned. "Are you sure he is okay?" *Why did she keep asking?* I wondered. She was making me anxious. "He is okay, thank you for asking," I said. When she left, I took Pepper's face in my hands. "You're okay, right, buddy?" I looked into his eyes. Actually, he did look tired, more tired than I'd seen him. Why hadn't I noticed?

Turning to Dennis, I said, "When we get home, we have to take him to the vet again." Pepper had been to several vets over the previous months because he'd had periods of lethargy and bouts of diarrhea. Nothing serious, we thought. Each veterinarian assured us that all was well. The last vet, right before the wedding, told us he had a stomach flu. "If you want to give him antibiotics you can, but I don't think it's necessary," he'd said. "I'll leave it up to you." I remember standing in the hotel room the next day, packing up to head to the castle, holding the antibiotics in my hand. I looked at Pepper. He seemed fine—we had just been on a long walk and his diarrhea had stopped. I didn't want to give him antibiotics if it wasn't necessary, worrying it would upset his stomach more. I contemplated it, and decided that since the vet said it wasn't necessary, let's not. I put the antibiotics in my toiletry bag. That moment—holding the antibiotics in my hand but choosing to put them away—would come to haunt me for the rest of my life. On the plane, Dennis tried to calm me down. "How many vets do you need telling you he is fine before you'll believe them?" Dennis said, a little frustrated. "But don't you think he's being awfully quiet?" I

asked. He paused. "I don't know. Maybe. No. He's Pepper!
He's just a good boy. Stop obsessing over bad things happening." I leaned back in my seat, trying to relax, but thinking,
*The thing is, I know now that bad things do happen. Two bad
things happened this year already.* I couldn't quite shake the
nagging feeling that something was wrong.

I was never so happy to get back to Aruba. We'd been away
for more than two months. It was late afternoon when we got
home and Quila and Laika, our two other dogs, were beside
themselves when they saw us. We took them all for a walk, and
as we went down our usual path along the north shore, I saw
Pepper stumble. Dennis saw it, too. Instead of heading up the
pack and running the fastest, the way he always did, he lagged
behind a bit. I slowed my pace to walk with him and he pressed
up against me and came to a stop. He was panting. "Okay, I
believe you," Dennis said, looking concerned. We decided to
take Pepper to the vet the following morning. A part of me
wanted to go right then, but only the emergency vet would
have been open and that was super expensive. That evening,
Pepper ate normally. He found an old toy and played tug-of-
war with Quila. I was relieved. *All is well*, I told myself.

We woke up the next morning with all of the dogs in bed
with us, as usual. When I wrapped my arms around Pepper I
noticed he was acting strange. He wouldn't look at me. I took
his head in my hands and stroked him and that's when I saw
that one of his eyes had turned blue. "Dennis!" I said. "Look at
Pepper's eye. It's blue!" Dennis was alarmed. "What does that
mean?" he asked. "Can he see?" I couldn't tell. "We have to go
to the vet *now*," I said.

As we headed to the car, I thought about my conversation with the flight attendant. I felt a twinge in my heart. *What if he is really sick and all this time we'd dismissed his symptoms because the vets didn't take them seriously?* I thought. I tried to not get ahead of myself.

We were the first ones at the veterinary clinic when it opened. The vet examined Pepper and ordered more tests. She asked if any of the previous doctors had tested his blood for tick disease. "Here in Aruba dogs get sick with it all the time," she said. "It's always the first thing we check for." I buried my face in Pepper's fur. How did I not think of that? Why hadn't I asked during previous veterinary visits if that test had been done? Had we been so caught up in planning the wedding and the honeymoon that I hadn't been persistent enough about Pepper's health?

The vet took a blood sample and returned ten minutes later with a grim look on her face. "This is one of the worst cases I have ever seen," she said. "His white blood count is so low, I honestly don't know how he is even standing up right now. And you say he went for a walk last night?" I was frantic. "He ran through the forest with me in Sweden just two days ago!" I cried. "We went paddleboarding last week. He is eating and drinking normally, too."

The vet said that Pepper had probably contracted the disease long before we went away. "This doesn't happen overnight," she said. "He is very, very strong not to have previously shown more symptoms than an upset stomach." I couldn't hold back my tears. "What can we do?" I asked. "We give antibiotics," she said. "It's all we can do. You have to come in every day for a shot and we'll see if we can get his blood count up. He needs to rest. No walks. I don't want to lie to you. This is not good." I looked at Dennis. His face was pale.

We drove home in silence. I couldn't believe what was happening. At home, we created a cozy space for Pepper on the couch. I fed him wet food and chopped up liver. He ate, which gave me hope.

On the third day, the vet was a little more optimistic, but Pepper was nowhere near out of the woods, she cautioned. "If things haven't improved by tomorrow, we can do a blood transfusion."

That night I took Pepper out into the garden. Just him and me. I tried to imagine what it must be like, suddenly not being able to see. *I did this to him*, I thought. *It's my fault. We shouldn't have taken him to Sweden. We should have seen one more vet. I should have asked for more tests. I should have given him the antibiotics.* I was consumed with guilt.

I could tell Pepper was scared. We walked a little and he pressed his warm body against mine. I told myself we would overcome this. Lightning strikes once, maybe twice, but three times in just a few months? No way. I squatted down to hug him and he leaned into me. My baby. *He trusts me. I'm supposed to take care of him—I'm his mother. How could I have let this happen?*

I started to cry. Sitting down in the dirt, I pulled Pepper into my lap and held him, or was it he who held me? I don't know. I looked up at the moon. Was it half-full, or half-empty? "Please save him," I said. I was speaking to Andrea. I hadn't asked anything of her since she died. People kept telling me she was an angel now, and that she'd always be by my side. If that was true, I wanted her to hear me now.

"Andrea," I said, my voice stern but calm. "I need you to help me. Help Pepper, please. I need him here. If you can hear me, save him. I'm counting on you. You owe me this." That last sentence sounded foreign to me. I sounded angry when I said it. I realized, I *am* angry. I needed her to save him. *If there is a God, a spirit, anything out there, I will wake up tomorrow and Pepper will be better*, I told myself. I was willing the universe to heal him. I felt that if I asked out loud, it would happen.

Before we fell asleep, I wrapped Pepper in a blanket by my feet. I didn't want him to be cold. When I kissed him good night, he barely lifted his head. I went to sleep holding him, repeating to myself, to Andrea, to God, to anyone who might have been listening: "Save him. Please, save him."

I awakened to a gasp but it wasn't mine. It was Pepper. He couldn't breathe. I called the vet in a panic. "Bring him in right now," she said. "Hurry." Pepper couldn't stand. We carried him to the car and I sat in the back with him, holding him in my arms. "Breathe, baby, breathe," I whispered. I couldn't see the road through my tears.

We arrived at the vet and he was put on oxygen. "He is dying," the vet said, placing her hand on my shoulder. "It is happening now." Tears streamed down Dennis's cheeks. He buried his face in Pepper's fur. *This is not just my loss*, I thought. *It is our loss.* Maybe it's even more Dennis's loss—Pepper was "his" dog. Pepper always slept at Dennis's feet. Dennis took Pepper to work every day; he was the skate shop dog. Dennis loved him more than anything.

"He is in pain," the vet said. "We can help him. Let him go."

I look at Dennis. He nods. It all happens so fast.

She leaves the room and now time is standing still. Pepper is still struggling, but his gasps are farther apart. His eyes are calm when he looks into mine. I am vibrating with love for him and I am sure he can feel it.

iloveyouiloveyouiloveyouiloveyouiloveyouiloveyouiloveyou. I repeat it like a mantra. It's flowing through me like a prayer. *iloveyouiloveyouiloveyouiloveyouiloveyou.* I am intensely present. The space between Pepper's breaths is getting longer. I breathe with him. Dennis is sobbing. I am calm still. We hold Pepper tight. I love him so much—is it even possible to love this much and to die this much? He is so loved. In the minutes that pass I remember my grandmother and her quiet passing; the space between her breaths that grew longer and longer until there was nothing left but space. This is nothing like that. It's violent, terrifying, horrible, awful, overwhelming, too much to bear. Pepper is gasping for air. He wants to breathe. He wants to live. His eyes are panicked. The vet comes back in with a needle and she puts it in his neck or maybe his arm, I don't know. It happens so quickly. Too quickly. The gasping stops. He is gone.

I wail.

Dennis tries to pull us together—it's over. We have to leave. We have to get out of there. There is a back door. We leave through it. We are in the car again and we turn the corner and I realize— we left him behind. "*Go back!*" I yell. Dennis pulls the car over.

"We can't leave him there! We have to take him with us." I don't know how we got in the car so fast. We are in absolute shock. Dennis turns the car around and goes inside and when he comes back he is carrying Pepper wrapped in a sheet. He puts him in the car. We drive home with our dead dog in the backseat. I feel like none of this is happening, none of this is real. We come home and it's like we're moving through mud; everything is happening in slow motion. We're here, but everything is blurry, hazy. Dennis takes Pepper from the backseat and puts him in a shaded spot on the stoop next to the house. The sheet is a little bit brown—he's pooped himself. "They said that happens when you die, the body releases like that," Dennis says. I have no idea how he knows that. I didn't know. I never before held someone as they died. Before this year I didn't know that a heart can stop and be restarted and stop and be restarted again or that blood smells sort of like fishing nets but not really or that our feet get cold before we die or that in the last moment there is poop. Time before knowing these things was another life entirely. A different life. One I long for, with all of my might. I don't want to be here. I don't want to be here holding my dead dog while thinking about my best friend's bloody dress and the hairs that grew on my grandmother's chin. I don't want this life. I really, really, really want to leave and just go be somebody else. But I can't. I am where I am.

Through tears, Dennis brings the other dogs out one at a time to say good-bye. Laika is very cautious—she sees him from afar and she stops wagging her tail immediately. She walks up slowly and sniffs him before turning around to look at us. It's like she's asking me, "What's happened?" I look into her eyes. *I killed him.* The thought is there without warning and once I think it, it etches its way into my soul. *I killed him. I killed him I killed him I killed him.* This is my fault. I had the antibiotics in my hand. I squeeze my eyes shut to rid myself of the memory. Dennis gets Quila but she doesn't want to go near him, it's like she doesn't recognize him as him. Maybe his soul has left his body so she doesn't know where to look. I don't know. She lies down at my feet. Finally Dennis brings Ringo out. He sees Pepper and comes running over and without hesitation starts licking his face and his mouth. When he doesn't move or respond he turns to us, eyes big. "What's wrong with Pepper?" he asks. "Doesn't he want to play?" "I killed him," I say, but it's silent. I know I can't ever speak those words out loud. "He loved you so much, buddy," I say instead. "We have to say good-bye now." Ringo crawls up in my lap. Dennis gets a shovel.

Turns out, digging a grave takes a long time. We live on the north coast of Aruba and the earth is rocky and firm. I get a new, clean sheet to wrap Pepper in. We put him in the earth. I bring his favorite toy, a stuffed animal bear, and tuck him in. It feels strange to wrap the sheet around his face—I want him to be able to breathe. But then I remember he won't do anymore breathing. We cover him with dirt and pack the grave tightly. I find a big white rock that we set as a gravestone and small white rocks to circle the grave. Once it's over we sit on the couch. I look at my watch. It's eleven o'clock, still morning, and we have already buried our dog in the backyard. My mom has texted me in our family group chat. Is Pepper better? she asks. I answer, No, he died. My phone starts ringing and it's ringing and ringing. I leave it and go back to bed.

Bad things come in threes. That's what I've always heard. So now that my best friend, my grandmother, and my baby have left me in just a few months, does it mean it's over? Or are there more catastrophes knocking on my door? I'd like to know who's running this show because I don't know if I want to be part of it anymore.

Pepper's death throws me in a way I'm not prepared for. Everything I thought I'd learned in dealing with the loss of Andrea was a lie. I feel like I've learned nothing. It pains me deeply to admit this, so I don't tell anyone, but it's the truth: Pepper's death hurts me more than Andrea's. In a way, it's like I have to deal with three losses wrapped up in one, but I can't tell anyone how much pain I'm actually in. Pepper was a dog and Andrea was a human being, but Pepper was my baby and I failed him and it's added a level of pain to my grief that I'm not in any way equipped for. Andrea was an adult—she drove the car. I was responsible for Pepper. He was counting on me to keep him safe and I didn't. Pain is worse when it comes with guilt.

I am angry—angry that Andrea didn't help me. Any faith I might have had—in God, in spirit, in the universe—any belief that there was a purpose to any of this, that it was taking me somewhere, that I was divinely guided and one day this would all make sense, has been crushed.

There is a second truth that I also don't speak out loud, maybe because I can't bear to hear the words. I feel like I killed

Pepper. Objectively, I know I wasn't solely responsible. He had seen so many veterinarians and no one knew what was wrong, so how could I be? But I was his mom. I should have known. If I hadn't been so preoccupied with other things, if I hadn't been so self-absorbed, I would have known. If only. Fuck "if only."

I scroll through my Instagram account, from the beginning; 120 weeks ago, when I would be lucky to get a couple of likes on a photo, up to the present. Pepper was in almost every single one. He had been with us through everything, every big moment in our lives. I was Dennis's wife, but Pepper had my heart and he knew it.

I get the urge to drink. To party, to dance, to be crazy. Patrick, one of Dennis's best friends, is on the island. He knows death like I know death—his father passed away just two weeks before Andrea. We go out dancing. I get drunker than normal. I'm drinking to be somewhere else. Every day I sit by Pepper's grave. The first night after we buried him I wake up in the middle of the night crying so hard, all the dogs start barking. Dennis tries to wake me up but I am too deep in my dream. When I finally wake up I'm gasping for air—I can't breathe. I realize Pepper is all alone outside in the dark. We are all in here where it's warm and cozy and he is out there all alone. Dennis keeps telling me it's just his shell, his body, he isn't there, but I can't shake it. I feel like we've buried him alive. I run out at two in the morning with Pepper's blanket, thinking that if I cover his grave with it, then he'll feel more held. He will be cozier. I stub my toe on a rock and when I get to the grave I've realized how crazy I'm being, so I just sit there and wrap myself up in the blanket instead.

The next night it happens again—I have nightmares so intense I can't wake up. In my dream Pepper is out there but we aren't letting him in. He is howling for us and calling for us but we left him out in the cold. Dennis tries to stop me but I run outside. I fall asleep on Pepper's grave and when I wake up Dennis is picking me up and bringing me back into the house. On the third night he gets angry. "This has to stop. You can't be out here. You have to come inside," he says, but I've lost it. I don't care about anything else. I don't care about Andrea or my grandmother or Dennis or anyone. I only care about Pepper and the fact that no matter how many blankets I bring out into the backyard, he will always and forever be cold.

I feel like we put the grave too far away from the house. I wish we'd dug it much closer. Right next to the grave is a tree, but it's been dead since we moved in. It's been three years and it's just a tiny, fragile little trunk of a tree branch; we don't know what it once was. I decide to plant things around his grave and put a little bench there so we can sit next to him without lying in the dirt. Dennis goes along with it, so we buy jasmine flowers and a little greenery and I find a bench I love, but it's too expensive. I find myself wondering about Dennis: Is there a limit to how many times he can pick me up off the floor? He's done it all year. All year I've cried, all year I've been in pain, all year he's saved me again and again. And now it's not my loss, it's our loss. Pepper was a big-boy dog, a little doofus, funny, with such personality. Dennis loved him more than anything. Am I not supposed to hold Dennis at night so he can cry, too? But he doesn't cry. And I'm losing it. I'm losing it all.

I buy a lantern that's windproof and every night at sunset

I put candles in it and bring it out to Pepper's grave. It helps. When I look over I no longer see cold, dark death but a little glimmer of light instead. The light makes me feel like he is less alone. I stop going out to the grave in the middle of the night. The dead tree by his grave has burst into life. It's remarkable, really. The morning after we buried him I came out to sit with him and doubled over crying, so I grabbed the tree trunk to hold on. When I came to, I saw four tiny leaves springing from it. One leaf for each year of his life. We've lived here for years and there has never, not once, been a leaf on this tree. We always assumed it was dead. Maybe it was. Maybe Pepper lives on in this tree.

A month passes and now it's absolutely blossoming—the branches hang heavy with greenery and it's so beautiful. Someone tells me it's an Aruban cherry tree. We call it Pepper's tree. He was only a dog and people tell me to move on—they don't understand how my life has ended because my dog died. I guess from the outside, in the light of Andrea dying and then my grandmother, it's hard for people to understand why now, suddenly, I'm losing it. And it's clear that I am. I can't keep myself contained anymore. I keep bursting into tears at gatherings, at the beach with our friends watching the sunset, when I'm teaching yoga, at the grocery store waiting to pay for my vegetables. I don't care. I've kept myself together all year and I just can't do it anymore. And every night I think about all the things I could have done that would have prevented this. I make a list in my head. It's titled "All the Things I Could Have Done for Pepper Not to Die" and it's getting longer every day.

I try to stay busy, but I can't keep up appearances like I

did before. I forget to answer e-mails, miss meetings, show up late for yoga class. I don't feel like washing my hair or putting on clothes in the morning. But we have prior engagements and I have a career that's suddenly blossoming and it's hard to explain to people that my dog died and I no longer want to do any of it. When I get too consumed with sorrow I try to move my body because I know it helps. I roll out my yoga mat, or if it gets really bad I put on my sneakers and I run. I hate running, but when your mind is playing the record of how you killed your dog over and over, you'll do anything to turn it off. One afternoon I'm home alone and Ringo is pawing at Pepper's grave, and every time I close my eyes I see him out in the street at night, scared to walk because he can't see, and it's just unbearable so I grab my shoes and I run. I run and I run and I run and on my way back, I have to cross a street where a pack of street dogs live. I drive by them every day and there is one that I know isn't very nice, but I never worried about them before. It's there now, the big white dog that always tried to bite at my tires, but now he comes with a whole pack. There are so many dogs and they are all coming my way. I'm in the middle of a dirt road and there is nowhere to go. The white one is showing his teeth and growling and the others turn toward me and now I'm surrounded. I back up because I'm terrified to run. I try to remember what you're supposed to do if you get attacked by dogs, but I don't know because I've never contemplated it before. Is it like a bear attack and you're supposed to pretend you're dead, or are you supposed to run? I don't have time to think of it because they are barking now and they are so close, all ten of them biting at my feet. The hair on their backs is standing up and their eyes are black and I'm so terrified I freeze. They are going to kill me. I know it. I say a prayer, thinking, *This is it*, because my back is against the wall and there is nowhere to run, and right then, two of them start snapping at each other and, suddenly, they're not after me anymore but a dog fight happens instead. It's a whirlwind of teeth and whines and aggression, but there is a window there for me to escape and I take it. I bolt, knowing they might run after me, there are so many of them. I run faster than I've ever run in my life, expecting to get bit any second. The bite never comes. I get to the front door and my hands are trembling so much I can't get the key in the lock. When I finally get through the door I collapse, crying so hard my body doesn't know how to cope with it. I can't breathe and I'm hyperventilating and now the dogs are inside me; the fear and the terror and the panic is coming from within and it's all closing my throat and I can't breathe. *This is dying*, I realize. *This is it.* I manage to grab my phone and call my friend Rose, because if I die I don't want Dennis to be the one to find me, and then everything becomes black. When I come to, Rose is there. My head is in her lap and she is stroking my hair and telling me to breathe and I'm convulsing and trembling and sweating but also freezing. I have my running shoes on and my face is streaked with dirt. I can barely breathe and for a second I don't know where I am. "It's just a wave, dushi," Rose says. "Breathe." I try to pull air down into my lungs but it doesn't quite make it there—it's as if it just gets stuck. Why can't I breathe? "You're having a panic attack, you're not dying. You can breathe. There is air. Inhale. Exhale." She is so calm, so calm, so steady. My rock.

I can't breathe, but she says there is air so I believe her. Rose always tells the truth. The next inhale I take breaks the barrier to my lungs and reaches my body. As I exhale something lets go and I cry. It's a soft cry now. I don't know what's happening. Then I remember. "The dogs. They tried to kill me." "Shhh, it's okay. Don't talk. Dennis is on his way." I stay quiet. Dennis eventually comes and as he picks me up off the floor I wonder how many times is one time too many, but when he unties my shoes and lays me in bed I realize: there no such thing as too many. He is always here. I drift off. When I wake up I hear Rose and Dennis talking to each other outside. One of them is crying—it takes me a little while to figure out that it's Dennis. They are worried about me.

I'm worried about me. I decide to try harder.

Time passes by like nothing has happened and there are days when I feel almost normal. But then a wave of grief will hit and now it's not just Andrea or Mormor or Pepper in a wave of grief—it's all three wrapped up into one. And it means that I drown in the waves. I can cling to the surface in the in-between, but when a wave of grief hits me now, it takes me under. I have my worst moment since Pepper died right after we come back from teaching a retreat in Bonaire. It's been almost two months since he died and grief is like that; it will trick you. I did a good job teaching and holding space for other people and I only cried in Savasana, not when I was teaching anything else, which is good because it means I kept it together and people didn't really know. We come back and I've been busy and haven't thought about death too much. Dennis goes to run some errands and I'm home alone and while cleaning the house, I find Pepper's collar. It's something that simple—I just find his collar. We took it off as soon as we found out he was sick and it must have been put with all the other dog stuff, because I haven't seen it or thought of it since. Holding his collar a wave of grief comes and it's so intense, so deep, I feel like I'm drowning. Normally in a wave I'd call someone, do something, find someone to help me stay afloat, but this one is just so big I can't see any light at all. I try and try but nothing works. I decide I need to get out of the house because maybe then I'll stop crying, so I take the dogs to the north shore to go for a walk, but it keeps getting heavier and heavier still. I try to focus on my breath, to bring my attention to something, anything to shift my state of mind, but I can't. I'm in too deep.

We get to a beach and there is no one there, so I let the dogs off their leashes and let them run. I sit down in the sand and I've stopped crying, but I feel nothing. I'm numb. I think about Andrea and how I'll never see her again, and my grandmother and my mother, who is going through a divorce now—she needs me but I can't be there for her. And I think about Pepper's collar at home and how he'll never wear it again and how that was my fault, and all of a sudden I'm standing up. I'm not thinking anymore, I'm just walking. I walk and walk and I don't stop until I'm waist-deep in the ocean. My sneakers are heavy with sand and water and the waves are pushing me around. It's hard to stand. I look out at the sea. It's rough. *I could just keep walking*, I think to myself. I could just walk out. Out of life. I could. I hear Ringo barking and, suddenly, I'm pulled back into the moment. If I died, there would be no one here to take the dogs back home. It's the one thought that hits me and it's enough for me to turn around and walk back to shore. *If I walked into the ocean and died, who would take the dogs home?* It was a very rational thought. And it saved me. As I walk back to the car, Ringo is at my feet and Quila and Laika are running ahead and they are so joyful. The clouds part a little bit. I realize I'm wet. My shoes are wet. Why was I in the water with my shoes on? I see myself from the outside looking in. Soaking wet, fully clothed, walking my dogs back to the car. *What a silly moment that was*, I think, and that was that.

When I get home the wave is gone but I'm still feeling a little numb. I tell Dennis later in the evening as we're preparing dinner, "I walked the dogs today and thought that maybe I should just walk out into the ocean and not come back." Dennis stops chopping the onion that's on the cutting board in front of him. "You did what?" "It was just a thought. I got wet. It was stupid, I changed my mind. There would have been no one there to take the dogs home." I say these words to my husband like I'm casually talking to him about my day or sharing something that happened at work, but what I actually said was "I thought about killing myself today." I don't realize what I've done until after dinner. Dennis is outside, on the phone. He is crying. Crying hard. He hangs up and comes back inside. His eyes are red. "Why are you so sad?" I ask. He turns to me with fire in his eyes. "Do you realize what you just said to me? Do you have any idea how worried I am about you??" He starts crying and he hugs me and it's so tight I can barely breathe, but not because I can't feel love but because I feel so much of it. His heart is beating against my chest and he is crying and crying and crying. I hold him. "I love you so much. Please don't ever do that again," he says between sobs, and now I'm crying, too. I hold him and his heart and there is so much life here, not just death. I've let death take up so much space it's literally almost killed me. As I stroke my husband's hair and hold him close I decide: enough. Enough death. It's time I come back to life.

I wasn't serious about not wanting to live, but I realized I needed serious help, and started reaching out to my friends and family more. The next time I felt a wave of grief coming, instead of closing off, I picked up the phone. Having someone there on the other end of the line made everything more bearable. I realized I don't need anyone to give me advice or to tell me everything is going to be okay. I just need someone to be there. I had so many people in my life, but little by little I had sealed myself off from most of them, thinking I was alone in my grief. When I started opening up more and asking for help, I found that, actually, I wasn't alone. I had so much to live for. Andrea and Mormor and Pepper dying didn't mean the end of my life—it meant the end of a part of it. I was learning how to navigate the world without them in it. I knew: there was no going back. I had to move forward.

One day, I was in Savasana at the end of class when, suddenly, I felt Pepper's presence. I'd experienced this with Andrea, too, but every time the feeling was followed by a massive wave of pain and an overwhelming longing for life to be different. It wasn't fair that she died at twenty-four years old and it made me angry at the universe. When I felt her presence in moments of silence, I hadn't been able to stay with it because my perception of what should or should not be clouded the experience and she'd disappear. In the beginning, that pain was so searing I thought I wouldn't be able to survive—that I would die from my grief.

Then my grandmother passed. I loved her deeply, but the pain over her death was entirely different. It hurt, and I knew I would miss her, but it was her time. She had a long, beautiful life and died surrounded by people who loved her. At least I got to say good-bye.

When Pepper died, it was in the worst way, not in peace, and not silently, but in pain, with us clinging to him, not wanting to let him go, unable to save him. Had we let him down? Did he wonder why we didn't do more? Why we didn't take care of him better? I felt so guilty. It was consuming me.

Then he came to see me in Savasana. It was so quiet and suddenly I felt his presence. Before I knew death I would always wonder what people meant when they referred to that feeling; how can you feel someone's presence when they are clearly not there? Well, now I knew. I was finishing a class, lying flat on the floor on my mat at the end of practice, and suddenly I just felt him. He was there, covering me like a warm blanket on a cool night. I didn't cry. I didn't feel the pain, or the what-ifs, and I didn't get the image of his agonizing death. Instead, I smiled. I saw him running on the beach—always the only one of the four to come right back to my side while we were walking. He wasn't sad. He was happy. He was nudging my hand with his head, saying, "Don't worry. I'm still here."

Later, I posted an ode to Pepper below a photo of Ringo and me during my practice:

Late night candle lit yoga with this guy on my mat the entire time. He digs himself beneath the blanket I use for Savasana and puts his head on my neck in Child's Pose. He wants to be so close. All the time. I think about Pepper who would put his little face on the corner of my mat but not more. He'd lie there, looking at me, my feet landing just centimeters away from handstand to Chaturanga. He never flinched. Trusted me blindly. But he stayed in that corner, never interfering. Like he knew, I needed space to move. I wrote that word just now, move, and my phone autocorrected to Love. I need space to love? I guess it must be true. I think of all the loves I have lost this year and I lose my breath a little bit, once again. Like it's new information. But maybe that's all it is. Death. A little space to love. Ringo is close and I love him. Pepper has given me space to love and in that space love grows. I hope he feels it, somewhere. My love is growing thanks to you Pep. I will never understand death. But I understand this moment. For that I am grateful.

Three deaths and they are all still here. I just have to be still enough to feel them.

15

TRUST

When I had reached almost one million Instagram followers, I was approached by a Swedish publisher to write my first book. The idea was to put together a collection of yoga poses, healthy recipes, and stories of wisdom and spirituality. The title was, predictably, *Yoga Girl*. It's a weird thing, writing a book. The lag time between finishing it and seeing it in bookstores is months, sometimes longer. *Yoga Girl* was published first in Sweden and then the United States, where it went on to become a *New York Times* bestseller. Most of it was written before the string of tragedies in my life, but even the last parts I had to write—the dedication and acknowledgments pages—don't mention Andrea or Mormor or Pepper. The pain of the loss was still too raw.

The book launched in November 2014 in Stockholm. Along with the publication came a book tour and classes and speaking engagements. It was on that tour that I fully began to realize the success of my career. Everywhere I went, huge venues sold out. Hundreds of people lined up to take photos with me every day. I spent hours after every appearance hugging people who came to see me.

Because so many people had followed my story on social media, my classes weren't as much about poses anymore as they were about healing broken hearts. "You're a poet," people said. "We love you." "Thank you." "You're such an inspiration." "You have changed my life." I had a hard time wrapping my head around it—I hadn't tried to do anything. I was just coping, and sharing my story. I didn't feel like I was doing something great. Most days, I was just trying to survive.

While my star was rising, my mom was getting a divorce. She had been with David for as long as I was with Dennis and I considered him family. They'd struggled for a while.

My mom had had a string of men, and in my book each one was worse than the last. When she met David, things quieted down and I'd hoped for the best. I so wanted it to be love and for her to be happy. Then again, her happiness seemed to always be fleeting, always followed by depression and sadness.

When my grandmother died, I'd been worried from afar about my mother, but didn't want to step too close. My curse had always been thinking I had to save her, but at that point, I was busy trying to save myself.

Since that moment on the beach when I wanted to walk out of life, and afterward seeing Dennis in such pain, something within me had shifted. I saw how always being the one to be picked up made it easier to give up and lie down. It wasn't until the moment Dennis broke down that I realized just how self-absorbed I had been in my grief. After that, I was committed to making sure that it was Dennis and me, together. I couldn't close myself off in my grief anymore, I had to let him in. I knew now that healing wasn't linear—it's not something you do one day and then you're done. I was going to have good days and bad days. The key was to have someone to talk to when the bad days arrived. To share what I was feeling. To have someone by my side. I wished I could have been that person for my mom during her divorce, but after everything I'd been through in the past year, I had nothing left to give.

My mom told me that she and David had been fighting a lot. That was no surprise. She'd been calling me in the middle of the night, crying and telling me what a bastard he was. During those times, I barely had the chance to digest what she was saying before she'd call again, excusing him by saying, "He didn't mean it," or "It was all a misunderstanding." I hated talking to my mother about her relationships. It always came with drama, and my fearing for her mental state. David was charming and good-looking and funny, but he was completely unreliable, and he drank too much. They both drank too much when they were together.

I don't know what the final straw was, but the end of their relationship scared me. In my eyes, David was the one who took care of my mother, relieving me of the responsibility and the worry that had haunted me for the first twenty years of my life. *Who would look after her now?* I wondered. Mom said she was fine and she'd be even better once they were officially divorced. I was doubtful, but I tried to be supportive.

Dennis and I went home to Sweden for Christmas that year

and, surprisingly, Mom seemed to be doing great. She looked happier than I'd ever seen her. She credited her girlfriends for her transformation. The difference between this breakup and all the others, she said, was that this time, whenever she fell into pits of despair, her friends were there to pick her up. For the first time in her life, she had real female friends and having their support made all the difference. Celebrating Christmas with my family was beautiful and quiet, but I longed for New Year's Eve and the new start it represented. Mom and my sisters followed Dennis and me home to Aruba to help us ring in the New Year.

New Year's Eve was exactly what I'd hoped it would be. Mom looked great. Her hair was bright; she was tan, and wearing new mala beads that sparkled. But it was what she told me that made the evening perfect.

She talked about the epiphanies she'd had, and how for the first time in her life she felt like she was on the right path. She had changed her Instagram name to @yoga_mum and shared revealing captions, similar to mine, about life and the lessons she was learning. She had finally started seeing a proper therapist, who had prescribed antidepressants. I was so happy to hear she was seeing a therapist and taking medication. For me, this changed everything. She was taking care of herself. She was supported. I allowed myself to be cautiously optimistic that she really was on the right path.

When she was finished telling me about herself, Mom asked how I was doing. I realized that she'd been standing on the outside looking in through all of the recent pain and loss in my life. I wondered if my pain scared her the way her pain scared me.

She asked me about Andrea, which she hadn't done much in close to a year since the accident. They'd never met, my mom and my best friend. I decided to take a chance and give her an abbreviated version of what I'd been going through. I didn't want to cry—I didn't want to fall apart. It was a relief, letting myself be vulnerable with her. Eventually, the conversation shifted back to her and David and the divorce. I told her that I worried it would set her back. "Everyone is waiting for me to crash," she said. "But what if there doesn't have to be one? What if, for the first time in my life, I allowed myself to be happy?" I decided to lay it all out. "It's hard to trust you when you say that," I said. I went on to tell her about my deep-seated fear that something bad would happen; that I hated it when she was sad, but it was even harder when she was happy, because then everything was so unpredictable. "You've never had a breakup that didn't almost kill you," I said. "I don't think I could take you not being okay right now."

I began to cry. My mother took me in her arms and held me. It felt so good. I felt like a child. She wiped away my tears with her sleeve and took my face in her hands. "You never, ever have to worry about me trying to commit suicide again," she said. "I promise you that from the bottom of my heart. You can trust me. Let me be your mom."

Hearing her words was like hearing the sound of prison doors opening. I had walked around with so much fear for so long, always worrying about whether she was happy, and what she might do if she wasn't, and now her words were setting me free.

That night I had the best night's sleep I can remember in years.

The next day, for seemingly no reason at all, I started to feel annoyed by my bracelets. I was on my yoga mat and they just seemed to be in the way somehow. It was strange. I had worn bracelets for nearly a decade and never before noticed them while I was practicing. My bracelets were a part of me. Some I bought on trips as mementos of my travels around the world. One was a gift from a lady selling fruit in Cape Verde, another from one of my trips to Spain. I had friendship bracelets with Andrea and my friends Olivia and Daniella, and many more from students. Three of my bracelets were ones that Andrea's cousin made for me for my wedding, with string from Andrea's braids. I could trace my past on my wrists. Thirty-something bracelets I never took off—not even in the shower. I was doing a bind in Malasana and I just couldn't get the right grip. It was time to take them off.

I knew that cutting off my bracelets would be like chopping off all my hair, except there wouldn't be anything left to grow back. I knew it would be a huge thing, but I needed a fresh start. A clean slate. New beginnings. New Year's Day was the time for letting go.

I grabbed a pair of scissors and walked out to Pepper's

grave. It was late afternoon and a beautiful day. Pepper's tree had grown lush and gave me some shade. As I sat down in the grass, I heard the leaves moving in the wind. I cried for a while and then I took a deep breath and started cutting them off, one at a time.

"So long, 2014. Welcome 2015. May the New Year bring us peace and joy and normalcy," I said as I cut through leather and string. "I want everyday happiness and everyday sadness, but no fucking death or trauma or crisis. And balance. Please, God, Universe, Spirit, whoever is in charge—give me balance. Please just allow me to watch some sunsets and travel a little and stay home and argue about the dishwasher and write and kiss and do yoga and be happy and sad and feel okay. Thank you."

When I got to the last bracelets, the ones made with string from Andrea's braids, I almost couldn't breathe. Suddenly it felt unreasonable, this letting go. I pleaded with her for guidance. "I've been wanting for this year to be over for so long and now I'm sitting on Pepper's grave cutting your bracelets off my wrist and I don't know if that's okay. Where are you? *Can you please just give me a sign?*"

At that very second, I heard a loud crash inside my house. It sounded like someone had fallen—Dennis? Mom? One of my sisters? I put down the scissors and ran inside. No one was there. I looked around, and the blood drained from my face. My altar had fallen. It had toppled over, with no one around, and everything on it was scattered on the floor. I have no idea how it happened, but I knew that if I'd been looking for a sign . . . This was it. I cleaned up the mess, wiped away my tears, then walked back outside and cut the last of the bracelets off my wrist.

Another lesson learned: Letting go means releasing the pain, not the love. When someone we love passes away, they're close enough to give us signs when we need them, but far enough away for new love to grow. Love never dies. Death is simply a wide, empty space to hold all the love left behind. Love always stays.

16
———

BREATHE

Later that January I took a combined work and girls' trip to Thailand. I was hosting a retreat in Koh Samui and brought my friends Olivia and Daniella with me. Before I left, I received a message from my mom saying she was going through a rough time. She was sad again. It hadn't been for long, just a few days she said. I wrote her back with words of support but without letting that old worry pull me in. I reminded myself of our conversation in Aruba earlier that month, and that she was getting professional help. I could be in Thailand, enjoying time with my girlfriends. It was okay for me to live my life.

Olivia and Daniella and I are lying on the beach one morning after breakfast. The sun is still rising, it's early and not too hot yet. We're discussing whether we should order fruit salads or some smoothies and I'm listening to Olivia speak when I hear my phone go off. A message has come in through Whats-App. I had been speaking to Dennis and checking in about his day—in a few days he is coming to meet me all the way from

Aruba—so I assume it's him. A minute or so passes and I'm still listening to the conversation, but something is left lingering in my mind about that message. I suddenly get a bad feeling; is Dennis okay? I excuse myself and get my phone from my beach bag. I don't have to unlock it to read the message. It's from my mom. Seeing it freezes my blood to ice in a split second. As I begin reading, time seems to stop.

> Darling, I am so sorry that I didn't make it. I have tried but I can't do this anymore. Please promise me you will take care of Hedda and Maia for me. I love you so much. I'm sorry. Mom.

I am so sorry that I didn't make it. I knew what that meant. I feel faint. Olivia and Daniella see my expression. "What's happening? . . . What's going on?" I can't speak. I call my mom's number. No answer. I call again. No answer. I call and I call and I call. There is no answer. She is not answering. I stand up. The panic I feel inside of my chest is so vast, it makes all the panic I have ever experienced all throughout the past year fade in comparison. I'm having an out-of-body experience. I call and I call and I call again. She is not picking up. I fear my chest is going to burst from panic. I don't know who else to call. My mother might have just committed suicide and I am a twelve-hour flight away. My sister Hedda is in the south of Sweden, where she is attending art school. Maia still lives at home with my mom. I call her. She picks up on the first ring. Her voice sounds happy and casual. I hear her friends in the background. She obviously doesn't know anything, and I don't want her to know the gravity of the situation. *I love her so much*, I think to myself. I have to pull this off. She can't know.

I force myself to sound natural, as if I'm just calling to check in. "Hey, honey, it's me," I say. My voice sounds normal. I'm pulling it off. I can see myself from the outside looking in. I'm in Thailand standing on a beach, calling my thirteen-year-old sister in Sweden to see if she knows that maybe our mother has committed suicide. The situation is so absurd I can't wrap my head around the fact that it's actually happening. "Hey! How is Thailand?" she asks. She sounds so happy. "It's great," I say. "Hey, have you seen Mom today?" I ask. "Yes," Maia says. "We had breakfast this morning. Why? Is everything okay?" "Yes, everything is fine," I say. "I just need to talk to her. Everything is good." "Okay," Maia says. "I'm hanging out with some friends. Should I tell her to call you when I'm home?" "Sure," I say. "By the way, when you saw her this morning, how was she?" Maia becomes quiet on the other end. "Sad," she says. "You know how she is. She made pancakes but she was sad." "How sad?" I ask. "Really sad. Crying. But she said it was okay that I went to see my friends." Maia sounds worried suddenly, maybe wondering if she's done something wrong. "Are you sure everything is okay?" she asks. "Everything is fine!" I say. "You have fun. I'll call you later."

We hang up. I call my mom again. Still no answer. I'm panicking now. I don't know who else to call so I call David. We haven't spoken since before the divorce. He picks up on the second ring. "Rachel," he says. "How are—" I cut him off. "David," I say. "Something is happening. I need you to listen to me very carefully. Mom has done something to herself. I don't know what it is or how bad it is but I need you to go over there right now." His voice sounds flat on the other end of the line. He doesn't believe me. "Rachel—your mom and I are divorced now, I'm at work, you can't just—" I cut him off. "*Now*. You need to go *now*." My voice is trembling. People are looking at me on the beach. I'm almost screaming. Something in my voice tells him it's real. "Okay. I'm on my way." "Call the ambulance," I say. We hang up. He works close by and I pray he was at the office and that he'll get there quickly. It's bad. I know it. This time, it's bad. It's real. I call her again. No answer. A few minutes later my phone rings. It's David. "I'm here," he says. "I'm at the door. She is not answering the door or picking up her phone. Maybe she's not home?" "She's home," I say. My voice is calm. I become acutely aware of the fact that I'm the only one who knows that something is really wrong. I am the only one in the world who knows what is happening and I'm powerless. I have to convince him. "Shama!" He calls her name. I hear him banging on the door. "If you're in there, open the door." Silence follows. "You have to get a locksmith. Get them to take the door down," I say. "I don't know, Rachel . . . She changed the locks after I moved out. Maybe she is out? You need to calm down." "She is *not* out!" I say. "She is there." I'm convinced. "Look through the mailbox. Do you see anything?" He is quiet for a while. "I see her shoes. Wait, Henry is here!" Henry is my mom's dog. She takes him everywhere. "Wait. I . . . I see her purse. Her purse is here. And her keys. And Henry. She is inside. Shama! Open the door!" I hear it in his voice now, he knows she is in there. I'm not alone anymore. "Call the locksmith. Do it now." He hangs up. An eternity passes. I walk out into the ocean. The water reaches to my knees. I hold my phone to my chest. None of this is happening, but I know it is. I'm in the ocean. The water is warm. I look up—white clouds are passing by the bluest sky. *My mom might be dead*, I think. My mom might be dead. My mom might be dead. I let that reality sink in and I see the entire world changing around me. I float out of my body, all the way up into the sky. I see myself in a world where my mom is dead, where this time she succeeded. Where this time she takes her own life. From above I see myself, standing in the ocean in my orange bikini. I look so young, almost like a child. My blond hair reaches almost all the way down to my waist. I'm clutching my phone, willing it to ring. My mom might be dead. If it weren't for everything that's happened in the past year, I wouldn't have let myself grasp the gravity of what might be my new reality. But in this life, in my life, I know that lightning doesn't only strike once. It strikes twice. Three times. Maybe even a fourth. My mom might be dead. *I won't be able to live without her*. It's not a thought but a knowing. Even though I've spent my whole life fearing it, life without my mother is completely unimaginable. If she's dead, I'll die. She has to live. I'm willing her to live.

A lifetime passes before David calls back, but in reality it's maybe ten minutes. When I pick up the phone he is crying and talking to someone else. "She is inside. My ex-wife. I don't know, she might have done something, I'm worried . . . Her daughter is on the phone, she is in Thailand." I hear other people in the background. They are tearing the door down. "The ambulance is here," he says. "And the locksmith. We are almost in." I hear a shuffle of people on the other line. A loud bang, people yelling. David is sobbing now. "Shama!" he says. "Shama!" His voice has cracked. "We're inside," he tells me. "I see her. I see her. She is here. She is on the bed. She's here. She's unconscious."

I stay on the line until they have loaded her into the ambulance. He hangs up.

I fall to my knees.

I don't remember how I got back to the hotel room but I am sitting there with Olivia and Daniella when David calls again. "She's alive," he says. I choke on my tears because the relief is so sudden. They get stuck halfway up my throat and just sit there. I cry and I scream but there is no sound. It's all silent. It's relief but it's all-consuming pain because I can't fucking believe that this is happening. Olivia and Daniella hold me. "She's in intensive care," David says. "How did she do it?" I ask, but I already know. "Half a bottle of vodka and an entire bottle of pills," he says. "It was close. It was really close." David isn't crying anymore. "I can't be here," he says. "I can't deal with this. These past months . . . you have no idea. I have to go."

I understand. This is not his problem now. They aren't married anymore. He doesn't want to touch this with a ten-foot pole. "Your aunts are on their way. When they get here, I'm leaving." "Thanks for breaking the door in," I say. "Thank you for making me," he answers. "I'm sorry." The line goes dead.

The next call is from my mother's sister Stina. She sounds weary. "She is sedated but stable," she says. "We are here. We're not leaving. Who is going to tell the girls?"

"I'll tell them," I say.

The only thing worse than having to tell my siblings our

mother just tried to commit suicide is the thought of someone else doing it.

I call Maia first. "What is going on?" she asks. "Mom hasn't picked up the phone all day." Maia says she is at her best friend Nike's house. I am glad she is there. I'd been worried that maybe she had gone home during the day to find the door shattered and remnants of pills and alcohol.

"I have to tell you something," I say. "Everything is okay, but Mom tried to kill herself today. She is okay—she is alive—but she is in the hospital . . . It has nothing to do with you, nothing to do with us . . ." I say these things, I try to soften the blow, but I know it's all a lie. How can you try to commit suicide when you have children waiting for you at home? Of course it has something to do with us. She's our mother. It has everything to do with us, but I don't want Maia to feel like this is her fault. I don't want her to live with my guilt. I don't want her to think what I know she is already thinking: *Mom was crying into the pancakes this morning. I shouldn't have left. I shouldn't have gone to meet my friends.* Of course she should have gone to be with her friends! Because our mother is a grown-up and we should be able to have a normal fucking day without worrying about her dying.

I tell Maia all those things—Mom is sick; she loves us; she is going to get better—at the same time thinking it is all bullshit.

Maia is quietly crying. Tears burn like acid down my cheeks.

"Stina and Lisa are going to call you," I say.

Maia would have to stay with her father. She hadn't seen him in months, but she had to stay somewhere. No one knows how long Mom would be committed.

I call Hedda next. Might as well rip off all the Band-Aids at once. I know it won't be an easy call. Hedda was always a sensitive child. Right now, she is probably the one who is closest with Mom. Sometimes she would spend a whole day on FaceTime with my mom so she didn't have to be alone. She answers right away.

"Hey, honey," I say.

"What's wrong?" she asks.

"Are you with someone?" I ask. I worry she is going to have an anxiety attack and don't want her to be alone.

"Yes," she says tentatively. "My roommate is here," she says. "Tell me right away. What's wrong?"

I don't want her to have to linger with uncertainty for even a second, so I tell her the news in reverse. "Mom is alive—she is okay—but she is at the hospital. She tried to commit suicide today."

"What?" Hedda asks, her voice soft, almost like a whisper. "She tried to what?"

"She's okay," I say again. "But she tried to kill herself. She is at the hospital now. The aunts are with her."

Hedda stutters in disbelief. "No. I don't believe you. She wouldn't do that," she says. "You're lying. I spoke to her last night." "I'm so sorry, honey," I say. She begins to sob. She sounds so little. I wish I could have been there to hold her. For a long time I just listen while she cries. It is awful—the cry of a child having her whole life torn apart. She cries quietly, full of disbelief. Every sob feels like a knife twisting in my heart. Hedda and my mother had been through a lot together. Mom had been Hedda's rock when she went through her periods of depression. She doesn't know Mom the way I do. Mom had been stable for her. I repeat to Hedda what I told Maia, but she isn't having it. Her sadness turns to anger. "She loves us?" she cries. "*Loves us?* What kind of a person tries to take their own life when they have children they love? Children who rely on them? She was just going to leave us! She doesn't love us!"

I don't have any answers. Hedda is a four-hour train ride from Mom. "Do you want to go up to Stockholm to be with her?" I ask. "I can buy you a ticket."

"Why would I want that?" she asks. "Go see a mom who doesn't want me? Who abandoned us? Who only cares about herself? No thank you!"

She asks about Maia. Her concern for her little sister makes my heart break even more. "She is okay," I say. "She's going to her dad's house. Call her. Maybe it's good that you guys talk."

I have one call left to make. My brother, Ludvig, is two years younger than me and he'd lived in LA for most of his adult life. He and our mother are close—as close as you can be when you live a thousand miles apart. We'd been through this before together—when we were little kids. He knew this pain.

I punch in his number on my cell phone and it goes to voice mail. *What was I thinking?* California was fourteen hours behind Thailand. It is the middle of the night there. The call would have to wait.

The second I hang up, my phone rings. Hedda is on the other end and she is wailing. She can't talk. I am thousands of miles away—I wish I could will myself to be there with her, to be able to take her in my arms. But all I have is the phone.

"Breathe," I say. "Breathe." I guide her the way I did my students. "Come back to the body," I say, trying to soothe her. "Inhale. Exhale."

It takes a good ten minutes for her to calm down enough to be coherent. We stay on the phone while she walks to the school nurse's office. When we hang up, I turn to the ocean and scream.

It was late afternoon in Thailand when Ludvig returned my call. He greeted me joyfully. "Sis! What's up! How is Thailand?" I got right to the point. "I have to tell you something," I said. "Mom tried to commit suicide. She didn't succeed. She's at the hospital. She's okay, physically. Mentally . . . I don't know."

Sitting with my brother's silence was more than I could bear. I didn't know what to do so I kept talking. He said nothing. I told him the whole story, starting with Mom's text to me—except I lied and said she'd included his name. She hadn't. Her text didn't say, "Take care of Hedda and Maia and Ludvig." She didn't mention him in what she must have thought were her final words to her children. In my mother's world, I was the caretaker, the one who rescued, and Hedda and Maia would need to be cared for if she died. I lied to Ludvig because, to me, not being mentioned seemed worse.

Ludvig was crying now. "Are you going home?" he asked.

"No," I said. "You?"

"No," he said.

When Ludvig and I wrapped up our call, I was so tired I had to lie on the floor.

I checked in with my aunts every day. Mom didn't want to talk to me. She was too sedated to talk, they said, but I knew better. My mother was like a child. She was too ashamed to talk to me.

On the third day after her attempt, she was moved from intensive care to the psych ward. My aunt called to tell me. "Do you want to talk to her?" she asked.

Yes, I wanted to talk to her. I wanted her to tell me she was sorry and ask if I was okay so that I could tell her that "*No I am not fucking okay*. My mother tried to commit suicide, and even though she didn't die, in a way it's like she did. She left me. Again. I am all alone. *I am not okay I will never be okay after this.*" I didn't say any of that.

Mom's voice sounded like someone else's. It was hoarse, like she'd smoked too many cigarettes. The hoarseness was from the tube they had jammed down her throat to pump her stomach.

"Rachel?" she said. "Are you there?"

"Yes," I said, trying to hold back tears. Hearing her voice was a huge relief—it was like a part of me hadn't fully believed that she was actually alive. I had saved her life. I knew she was in pain. I knew that no matter how hard I tried, I would never be able to put myself in her shoes. I had never known despair that intense, suffering so deep that it made me want to leave this life. I should have felt sorry for her but I didn't. I was tired of feeling sorry for her, of worrying about her. I wanted her to worry about me now. I was her daughter and she was my mother—not the other way around. I wanted her to tell me she loved me, that she was sorry, that she was never going to leave me again.

"Where is David?" she said instead. It was like she'd slapped me hard in the face.

"What?" I asked.

"Where is David? Have you spoken to him? He isn't here. He isn't at the hospital."

I could scream into the phone and you wouldn't hear me, I thought. I didn't exist to her.

"Can you believe that I'm at the hospital and David still hasn't come?" she asked, sounding distraught.

"I don't know why David hasn't come, Mom," I said. "I'm in Thailand, remember?"

"Oh. Right," she said. "I have to go now."

My aunt got on the phone.

"Has she even asked about us?" I asked. "Has she asked if we are okay? Even once?"

Stina didn't answer the questions. "She is very confused," she said. "This has triggered something deep within her. You know this is not about David. It's about her pain. She loves you. More than anything."

I felt sick. "She has a funny way of showing it," I said.

Stina tried to comfort me, but her effort was in vain. My mother had tried to commit suicide, and after saving her life, and three days of silence, I finally got to talk to her and what did she say? She asked about David. She didn't ask about me, or my siblings, or whether we were okay or safe. The only thing that mattered to her was that David wasn't there.

At some point in our lives, whether we like it or not, we are going to find ourselves face-to-face with the very thing we fear the most. That's the thing about fear; we can't ignore it. It guides us to all the places we are trying to avoid and we can't escape it however hard we try. We try to keep our fears at a distance but they stay within arm's reach; close enough to maintain the ideas we have of ourselves but far enough away to pretend they don't affect our lives. But they do.

I was faced with a fear that week I never in a million years thought I'd have to encounter. Still, I was expecting it. Somewhere deep inside I knew it was coming. My heart had been trembling with terrified anticipation, waiting for this moment to come for more than twenty years. It happened. My entire body was stiff with shock. Everything hurt. But I was alive.

A few days later I was sitting on a small wooden deck, trying to write and process and meditate. I felt like my heart had been thrown into a washing machine—I didn't know which side was up anymore. In the scope of a few months I'd had surgery, lost my best friend, lost my grandmother, buried my dog, and almost lost my mom to suicide. As the sun rose, I wrote in big letters across the page: "IS THERE A REASON THIS IS HAPPENING TO ME?" The pain sitting inside of my chest was so big for a moment, I feared it would suffocate me. It was unbearable—I couldn't take it. Out of all the moments of pain I'd experienced throughout the past year—and there had been so many—this one was one of the worst. I felt something worse than sadness; I felt numb. My heart was a big, cold empty space. Suddenly, the deck was filled with specks of light. It was everywhere; tiny glimmers of light glittering across the wooden floor. Immediately, I pulled a deep, full breath all the way into the bottom of my lungs. As I exhaled, I looked out at the ocean. The first rays of the sun were rising from the horizon and were hitting a wind chime hanging in a tree branch above me, illuminating the deck. This was the light that had followed me since Andrea died. The light I'd seen again and again, during my most challenging moments. I put the pen down and sat in quiet meditation for a long time, allowing the numbness to stay as it was. I reminded myself that the biggest pain always came from resisting it. I took a deep breath, feeling it all. When I opened my eyes the sky was a warm orange, golden clouds passing above me. It was one of those sunrises that stay with you; a remarkably beautiful one. I stayed there for a long time, letting the light warm my skin. I picked up my notebook again, looking at the sentence I'd just written across the page. IS THERE A REASON THIS IS HAPPENING TO ME? What if this wasn't happening to me, but for me? What if there was a purpose, a reason for all this, somewhere? I wasn't sure, but I had to believe it. I had to hope.

The little girl within me whispered, "Soon, we'll be grateful for this."

17

____

FEEL

Dennis met me in Thailand and we flew to Costa Rica for Envision Festival 2015. A year had passed since I'd been there with Andrea. I was nervous about reliving our time together, but happy to be back in my second home.

Last year when I was there my social media accounts were just beginning to take off and now I had a team traveling with me. Besides Dennis and Ringo, my friend Rose joined us as well as Ben, the photographer who'd been with us all around the world over the last year. I'd gone from "that yoga teacher" to "Yoga Girl" and it seemed as if half of the people at the festival had found their way there from my posts.

I wasn't just living with my heart on my sleeve—I was living with my heart on the Internet. People knew the most personal aspects of my life. I walked up to the ticketing office and the whole line went silent. I overheard a group of girls whispering. "That's yoga girl . . . OMG, did you hear what happened to her? . . . I think she is teaching on Saturday." We went to grab food at the local market and a girl pulled out her phone and snapped a photo of me without even asking. It felt like a violation and I decided to address it. "Hi!" I said, walking up to her and her friends. "How are you?" My voice was angry. I was expecting them to be cocky, to pretend like they hadn't just taken a photo of me without my permission. The girl holding the phone looked at me, her eyes tearing up. "I'm so sorry!" she said. "I love you so much. You are my biggest inspiration. I didn't think you wanted to be bothered here with everything that has happened this past year, but I just wanted to remember this moment. I'll delete it."

I almost cried. There was a part of me that still didn't understand why I was getting so much attention. People related to my very human struggles. I put it all out there and they really did care. I felt myself soften. The girl didn't have bad intentions. "Let's take a proper picture instead," I said.

I took a few photos with the group. They were thrilled.

"We came here from Connecticut to take your class," the girl said.

"You are going to love Costa Rica," I replied. "It's so beautiful here."

The girl nodded. "I'm just excited to take your class," she said. "It's the center of our trip. We wouldn't have come here if it weren't for you teaching. Can I hug you?"

"Of course," I said.

We embraced and when she let me go she was crying. "I lost someone, too," she said. "Thank you for putting into words everything I could never say."

The moment with that girl could have turned out so differently. I had learned a valuable lesson from her. After that, I looked around with loving eyes at the people at the festival who recognized me, rather than feel like an animal in a zoo. Through yoga and social media, I was building a community of people who had been through pain and loss. I had touched people I would normally have never had the chance to meet. And they touched me.

This moment is the perfect teacher, I wrote on Instagram. Notice the signs and how the universe speaks to us all. There are not wrong turns. Everything is exactly the way it is supposed to be.

Sometimes I felt that if I'd just repeat it enough, eventually I'd actually believe it.

My mom decided to come to Costa Rica while I was there for the festival. *Why?* I wondered. We had barely spoken in the month since her suicide attempt. I didn't want her to come. Costa Rica was my place—my country. It was how I escaped her in the first place. And now she was coming here?

The little girl inside of me wanted to see my mother. The grown-up me wanted to say, "Go to hell! You're too fucked up. I'm done dealing with your shit." I didn't say any of that.

We decided to meet at a café we knew in Dominical, which was a short drive from the festival. I knew I was harboring a lot of anger toward her, but I didn't know what to do with it. She was in the process of "healing," she said, so I couldn't direct it at her. I had never known how to be angry with my mother.

We hugged. Actually, she hugged me. I couldn't respond. I just stood there stiffly. Dennis and Rose filled in the silence with small talk. I feared that if I spoke I would start to cry, and I didn't want my mother to see me sad.

"How has the festival been so far?" she asked. "Was your class nice?"

In spite of myself, I told her about something that happened the night before—a terrible situation involving Andrea's boyfriend, Gabriel.

Driving to the festival to see one of our favorite bands, I got a phone call. It was Gabriel's mom. I knew him well, but I'd never spoken to his mom before. "Have you seen him?" she asked. I hadn't, not since the day before. He was supposed to stay with us but had changed his mind last minute. "I got a strange phone call from him and now I can't reach him. I'm worried. He hasn't been himself since . . . since the accident." "I'll look for him," I said. "I'll call you as soon as I see him." I told everyone to keep their eyes and ears open. We didn't have to look for long. Walking through the main gates, we heard a commotion. A big crowd had gathered around whatever was taking place. There was lots of noise. We didn't give it too much thought, but then suddenly I heard someone scream. *I know that voice*, I thought. *I know that scream*. Dennis asked someone in the crowd what was happening. Some guy was tripping out, they'd said. It had been going on for a while.

I walked closer, fearing the worst. "Andrea!" the voice cried. "Andrea!" I started to run, elbowing my way through the crowd. "Let me through! I know him!"

Gabriel was on the ground with five big men holding him down. I barely recognized him. His eyes were wild and he was foaming at the mouth. He was strapped onto a stretcher. "Rachel!" he cried when he saw me. "Macha! Help me!"

People were staring and making comments. "That guy is fucking nuts" . . . "Tripping his fucking balls off " . . . "Psycho."

I squatted down next to him. His chest was heaving and he looked panicked. I asked one of the EMTs what was happening. "He is having some sort of episode," he said. "We believe it's drug induced. He was hurting himself and when his friend tried to stop him he went for him."

I turned around and saw Luigi standing there. "What happened?" I cried. "I don't know," Luigi said. "He lost his mind. He was hurting himself, kicking himself. I tried to stop him. I don't know what he is on. But he flipped and tried to hit me. It took so many people to hold him down. We had to call the ambulance." Luigi almost started to cry. "He was crying for her," he said. "For Andrea. Screaming for her. Again and again."

I watched as he was loaded into an ambulance. I couldn't let him go alone. As I climbed into the rig, an EMT ordered me to leave. It was against regulation, he said. I refused to budge, pushing my boots up against the ambulance door for leverage. "Please," I said. "His girlfriend died. That's what is happening to him. She was my best friend. There is no one else here for him." I saw a glint of recognition. "She had an accident?" the man asked. "The one they sent to the wrong hospital?"

I nodded. He knew. Everyone did. It had made national

news. Afterward, every hospital in the capital held emergency meetings to implement new rules mandating that residents were no longer allowed to be in charge of emergency room admissions. "Yes, her," I said. "This is her boyfriend." The EMT nodded. "Okay," he said. "You can stay."

I held Gabriel's hand for the long ride. I had hardly seen him since the days after the funeral—he barely returned my texts. I had heard from Andrea's family that he was in bad shape. As I looked at him lying there, my heart ached. He was sick with grief over Andrea. I could only imagine what it had been like for him. She was the love of his life. He'd been there with her. He'd ridden with her in the ambulance as the life drained from her body. For a second I remembered the overwhelming guilt I felt when Pepper died, holding his lifeless body in my arms, feeling like I somehow could have prevented it. I remembered feeling so numb, thinking about walking out into the ocean and not coming back. I could not for a second begin to imagine what this past year had been like for Gabriel. Maybe he was blaming himself for not being able to save her. Maybe the guilt was eating him alive. His chest was still heaving, but he was beginning to calm down.

"Does he have to be strapped down like this?" I asked the EMTs. No one answered. Finally we got to the hospital. Juliana, Andrea's sister, arrived and I was relieved to have her take over. "I got this," she said. I went back to the festival, and it wasn't until now, telling the story, that I realized how traumatic the whole thing had been.

As I told my mom the story, I began to cry. My mother moved close and held me. If only she hadn't spoken. "Why are you always the one fixing these situations?" she asked. "Who made you the savior? It wasn't your job to get into that ambulance. You have one job and that is to take care of yourself."

I didn't know whether to laugh or cry. It had only been a month since she'd sent her suicide text telling me to take care of my little sisters. Her children. I had been taking care of her since I was a little kid. Who made me the savior? You did, I wanted to say. You're the reason I'm like this. I stayed quiet and pulled away from her embrace. Her words had cut me like a million shards of glass. We were never going to be okay.

18

SHARE

I only had a few days at home in Aruba before I was off again, this time for my biggest tour yet: the Happiness Tour. My book debuted in the United States in late March and I was committed to do a twenty-seven-stop tour with huge classes, press events, and book signings. It kicked off in New York and lasted through mid-May. As grateful as I was for my success as Yoga Girl, for the millions who joined my Instagram account, for the thousands who had come to my classes, I missed Dennis and our puppies and I longed for quiet nights in my own bed.

Life on the road was hard. The days were long and I never got enough sleep—rushing from meetings to interviews to airports to car rentals to yoga classes to hotels to more airports. My body was aching for routine. Rituals helped to keep me grounded and sane. I traveled with crystals and gems, my angel cards, and palo santo.

I posted on social media three times a day. It helped me to feel connected. Sometimes I thought I had to be crazy, baring my soul on such a superficial platform that seemed only to care about Kardashians and thigh gaps and discounted weight loss teas. Everyone tried so hard to show how perfect their lives were with Photoshopped pictures and stories to match, and there I was, telling more than two million people about my pain. But then I thought, *There are people out there who long for the relief of knowing that others feel pain, too.* Instagram doesn't have to be a highlight reel of all the things we fear we are not. It can be more than perfect angles and perfect bodies and perfect food and perfect lives. It can be real. Human. Raw. It can be a companion for lonely moments, to remind us we are not alone. It was for me.

When the Happiness Tour ended I traveled to Europe for more signings and classes. Sweden was on the schedule and Mom insisted that Hedda, Maia, and I meet with her to talk.

We all met in the lobby of my hotel. Five months had passed since her suicide attempt and she hadn't had a proper conversation with any of us about what happened. The only thing she had told us was that a few days earlier, she was feeling good and decided she didn't need to take her antidepressants anymore. So she stopped. She didn't tell anyone. A fight with a loved one sent her over the edge into a pit of depression and she couldn't climb out. That's all she shared.

She didn't explain anything more than that and the conversation began and ended with her, how she was having such a hard time and she'd always had a hard time and poor her. Her whole life had been poor her, and normally I would sympathize, but I just couldn't do it anymore. I was sick of her being a victim, of her being so fragile. I was done with it. We started to argue. She accused us of not being supportive of her. We were shutting her out. We had our own clique. My sisters and I looked at one another. Damn right we did. We wanted answers, support. Maybe it was still too sore, too painful, but she didn't want to talk about any of it. Instead, she talked about what good friends she had and how supportive they were, and she still wasn't taking antidepressants, or seeing a therapist, but she was taking vitamins and drinking green juice, and getting some sort of treatment for her adrenals, she said. She could do this on her own. It would all be fine!

I saw red. "You need to be on medication," I said. "At the very least, you need to commit to seeing a professional. I am not going to trust you—we are not going to be able to trust you—until you have professional help." My mother refused. She had had an awakening, she said. This time was different. She could take care of herself.

I had heard that story so many times I wanted to vomit. If all it took for us to feel secure, for us to be able to heal a little more, was for her to commit to seeing a therapist, was that too much to ask? *Is that too big of a commitment to your children? The children you were so willing to abandon?* I couldn't comprehend it.

"Go for us," I implored her.

"I'm done doing anything that isn't for me anymore," she said. In a big way, I recognized that feeling. Were we all having a similar awakening, but on two opposite ends of the spectrum? Hedda broke down crying. I knew what she was thinking. What happens the next time she gets sad? The next time she cries? What then? Will we have to live like this forever—wondering when our mother might kill herself? Why doesn't she want to get better?

Mom stood and walked out of the lobby, leaving me with Hedda under one arm and Maia under the other. Both were crying. I had had enough. If my mother wasn't willing to give of herself—not even to her own children, who were suffering—I was finished protecting her.

I went back to my hotel room, picked up my phone, and logged into my Instagram account and started writing.

> July 17
>
> My name is Rachel and I am not ok. I haven't shared this properly before even though I always share most of everything but in February of this year, my mom tried to commit suicide. It shattered me on a level so profound; I've lost my sense of identity. She abandoned me and it's not the first time and now our family is in a million pieces.
>
> When it happened, I'm five years old again but this time it's not after my birthday party, it's during a trip I took to Thailand and she is in Sweden. It's not her fiancé crashing his plane into the ocean but her husband divorcing her. It's not suicide letters neatly left in sealed envelopes, one for me, one for my brother and one for everyone else, it's a message through WhatsApp and she is telling me to take care of my sisters and my brother and she's so sorry she didn't make it. It's still vodka and enough pills to ensure a certain death.
>
> The last time, it was my grandmother calling the

ambulance. This time it was me in a foreign country, on the phone with her ex-husband and the locksmith and the police, trying to explain that they NEED to knock the door down because my mother is dying she is almost dead it's for real I promise but no one will believe me. No one will believe me but they do as I say because I'm hysterical. It takes forever and time has frozen but they do as I say and they screw the bolts out of the door and the ambulance comes and she is unconscious on the bed and the whole time all I can think is how will I ever live without my mother when she is the center of everything. And now it's five months later and nothing has healed. No one is fine and I am so angry I want to scream until my voice is gone and I'm sad and I'm scared and I'm five years old wondering if it's all my fault. Maybe I should have been better, less fussy, teased my brother less. Maybe if I am perfect my mom will want to live. So I become perfect and my entire life revolves around being the best at everything and suddenly I'm 26 and history repeats itself and people tell me "it had nothing to do with you" but how could it not have anything to do with me when I am the one always saving her life?

I had never shared that part of me before on social media. I'd kept it to myself because I was afraid of upsetting my mother and it was growing inside of me like a cancer. I didn't know if what I had done would upset her, or if she would feel it was like a betrayal. All I knew was that putting it out there was a huge relief. Some people commented that I was jeopardizing her recovery, and that her personal story was not mine to share. Maybe they were right, but I didn't care. I was angry. This was my story, my life, too. Since Andrea, I had shared every heartbreak, every loss, every moment of pain through Instagram. It was a critical part of my healing journey and I wasn't about to stop now. It didn't matter what my mother thought. I was done walking on eggshells around her.

My mom texted her response: I would have appreciated you asking me first before sharing that online. But it's alright. I love you. We are going to get through this.

I didn't know it yet, but we had just taken our first steps toward healing. My mom was doing this in her own way, and for the first time in my life . . . so was I.

19

___

CREATE

Dennis wanted a baby. He had wanted a baby since the wedding, but I was too busy—or too terrified to try. I kept waiting to feel whole enough, to be healed enough, for something as monumental as motherhood. The shaman in Costa Rica had said I'd never pass on my pain—or the pain passed down from my ancestors—to my child. My daughter, he had said specifically. That was my purpose in life; to transform that collective familial pain and let it go. I deeply believed that to be true. From the time I was a little girl I'd said I wouldn't have a baby until I was "done." Healed. Happy. I didn't want to do what my mom had done—have children in the midst of so much struggle. It's what most people do; we can't help it. We can't control what comes our way, and when we are faced with loss and adversity, we do what we have to do to survive. I knew that what had happened in our past had to be, or I wouldn't be here. I tried to put myself in my mom's shoes; pregnant at twenty years old, living through so much trauma and loss, being a single mom. She had moved mountains for us. I had so much compassion for my mom—I loved her more than anything, and for as long as I'd lived she was the most important person in my life. I knew she had done the best she could. But her way was not my path. I was still angry at Mom and needed to focus on myself. But somewhere deep inside me, a dream was forming. A dream that involved a baby, and all of us being a family.

Yet I was still wounded. Broken. I wanted to be a mother at some point, but I could feel there was still a piece missing inside of me. In the meantime, I focused on our business. We had created so much in such a short time, and Dennis and I now ran several companies together. I'd taught classes of more than a thousand people. Launched a huge online platform. Started two nonprofit organizations. Written a *New York Times* bestseller. *What else could I do if I put my mind to it?* I wondered. A yoga studio. That would become my next goal. There was little yoga in Aruba, and the community I'd built dispersed when I started traveling so much. I yearned for a home base, a place to set down roots, a place where I could work from home.

I drew up a business plan for a studio I called Island Yoga. Dennis and I started looking at local properties. Things were moving. We found a property and took a loan. The place was a ruin and we'd have to tear most of it down, but we had the keys in our hands. There was a big open space, with a beautiful wood-beamed ceiling, and I envisioned us one day lying on yoga mats looking up. Island Yoga was coming true.

I told Dennis one day over dinner that once we'd had the studio up and running for a year or so we could "sort of, kind of, maybe" start thinking about one day having a baby. Construction was scheduled to begin in the spring of 2016. With luck, the studio would open before my twenty-eighth birthday. Maybe the year after that, I said.

Some people thought I spent all day at the beach or on my yoga mat. That was far from the truth. I wasn't just Yoga Girl from Instagram anymore; I was Yoga Girl, business owner, boss, CEO, chairman of the board. I was running four businesses in three countries, hosting retreats, teaching workshops, touring, managing social media, doing animal rescue work, all the while trying to stay present in my community. It was an enormous amount of work and there were moments when I felt dizzy just thinking about all of it. And it turns out, building the largest yoga studio in the Caribbean from the ground up wasn't a walk in the park! Construction was extremely stressful, and we ran out of funds more times than I could count. A few months into planning for the studio I started feeling overwhelmed. My mind and my body were always busy. Everything was nonstop. I loved the go-getting side of me (because of it, I'd manifested more magic in one year than I could have ever imagined!), but I was longing for rest. I just didn't know how to slow down.

The stress of dealing with business partners, construction setbacks, and long yoga tours was taking a toll on me. I decided I needed time for myself. For more than eight years, I'd wanted to attend an annual meditation retreat called Path of Love, but it had never been the right time. Every time I planned to go, something had gotten in the way—another trip, work, life. But the seed that had been planted long ago started sprouting.

I didn't know much about Path of Love, except that it was billed as a deeply transformative healing retreat. I'd heard about it when I was eighteen and participating in my first ever retreat, the one that would come to forever change my life. It was eight years later, and I just knew it was time for me to go. The last time I had done a group like that it had spurred me to leave Sweden and start on a whole new path. It had changed my life in the most magical of ways. I felt ready to dive in once again. I e-mailed, asking if they had space left in the May group in Germany. They responded that yes, they would love to have me. At least I had a few months to prepare, and Envision Festival in between.

At the end of February I returned to Costa Rica for Envision, this time with Olivia. It was hard to believe another year had passed, two since I'd been there with Andrea. *How does time work?* I wondered. *Is it linear? Is it all layered together and stretched out and mushed up into one weird experience?*

It was the first time I'd felt like myself at the festival since Andrea died. The previous year everything was too raw, too sad. I tried to channel her but I couldn't do it. This year I saw her everywhere. Her hair, her earrings, her smile. Her spirit was omnipresent. She was as alive in this community as she had ever been. Dancing. Bartering with vendors over twenty-dollar skirts. Sneaking up on people to tickle them. Losing her car keys again and again. Rolling out her yoga mat, wondering which side is up. Laughing. Always laughing. I saw her and I felt her.

After one day at the festival, I was bursting with gratitude. What better recipe than yoga and dirt and sweat and tears and hugs and so much love. Everywhere I went, people stopped to hug me. Complete strangers gave me gifts of fruit and crystals.

A woman offered me a Thai massage. Normally I wouldn't have accepted, but as I was saying no, it hit me: *Why not say yes? Why not just let yourself receive?* So I did.

It was dusk and I lay down on some blankets under a tree. I don't know how long she worked on me but my whole body was buzzing. She finished at the crown of my head and when she left, I felt Andrea's hands take over. It was so real. I felt her, heard her, smelled her. She was sitting behind me, her palms pressing on my crown and third eye. She was humming and I was crying. For the longest time we stayed like that. Olivia and Laura came over and held me and then it was the four of us, wrapped up in a ball of love and tears and the kind of friendship you can't put into words. They felt her, too.

I had a major insight. It was safe to relax. It was okay to receive. Andrea made that happen. She sat with me to help me understand I needed to let love in. All I had to do was stop resisting. I shared the realization with my online community: The universe wants to hold you. Please let it.

My mom had been texting me almost every day. I miss you, she said. How are you? Do you need something? I rarely responded because I didn't know how. During my practice that week, I started playing around with variations of King Pigeon. The pose is demanding and I'd struggled with it my whole life, but it was suddenly available to me. I hadn't been practicing it, or fighting for it, or struggling to deepen my practice. It just happened. Maybe my heart was finally open enough for the pose to find me. After I'd finished Savasana I rolled up my mat, reached for my phone and texted my mother back. I miss you, too.

It had been a big two weeks in Costa Rica, with lots of

opening, cleansing, and healing. I still felt Andrea so closely, but it was a different kind of feeling. It wasn't as painful anymore. I missed her, but I had finally stopped waiting for her to come back. I didn't have to call her cell phone, hoping she would answer. She was already there. She was everywhere.

I flew home to Aruba on the second anniversary of Andrea's death. I could have changed my flight and stayed in Costa Rica for another day, but I didn't. Instead, I was back home in Aruba, sitting on a rock in my garden, watching the dogs play and wondering if it was going to rain. I always felt closer to her when it rained.

I had come to terms with the fact that I was broken. Not in a sad or bad way, but in an it-is-what-it-is kind of way. Life happened and I adjusted accordingly. We're all a little bit shattered. Pain and heartache come our way and with time we develop patterns that we think will protect us. But that only keeps us in fear.

There are traits in me that aren't necessarily a part of who I am, but fallouts from what I've seen in this lifetime. For instance: I will probably always have a huge fear of abandonment. It stems from my parents' separation when I was two, my stepfather's death when I was four, my mother's suicide attempts, and every divorce, trauma, and death I've experienced since. As a result, I have to be mindful of what's real and what's fear.

I'm scared of being left out. I'm controlling—I want things to happen my way, and I often assume things are going to go wrong if I'm not in charge.

I micromanage everything. I expect people to fail me,

or disappoint me, or leave me, so they often do. It has been instilled in me since I was a little girl that if I don't do it, none of us will survive.

I don't trust easily, and I don't give second chances.

I'm messy. I'm emotional. I love hard and hurt over little things. I take everything personally. I want to fix everyone, even if they're not broken.

I want the world to be whole because that means I am whole.

So much of how I feel and act is connected to the past. Part of my journey is figuring out what is truly a part of me, what brings my light out into the world, and what is baggage masquerading as personality. What is action, and what is reaction? Am I moving with love or with fear?

I have learned now that the only way to make peace with who you are is to make peace with your past. Explore all of it. It brought you here and it made you who you are; but is this you at your fullest potential? Do you see love in everything? Is this your purpose? Ask questions. Peel off the layers. Notice the signs.

The more I reflect on experiences, emotions, and thoughts and how they relate to my past, the more in touch I feel. I understand, more and more, that absolutely nothing is random. Everything is perfectly orchestrated to bring us what we need to elevate our being. To live out our purpose. My purpose here has to do with healing, with moving others through trauma and grief, with inspiring acceptance and kindness and fearlessness. It has little to do with photo shoots and business meetings—but that is my way of getting there. It comes with the job.

For so long I wondered, What is the point of all this? I am finally starting to get it. I feel butterflies flutter in my stomach when I think of the true potential of what lies ahead. I am going to change the world. I know I am. I've spent my life so far working through pain and trauma to get here. To understand that I am in the business of teaching and promoting love.

I shared my thoughts on Instagram: I feel like I am on the cusp of something big; as a teacher, as a student of life, as a human being. This is the path. I'm uncovering my true dharma and it's making the earth rumble beneath my feet. I've made a decision: next month I'm going away. For a while. From everything. Into myself. Back to basics. Will share more soon. All is well.

20
—

HEAL

I spent some time in Sweden before heading to Germany to attend Path of Love. I stayed with my mother and Maia, who was now living there again. It had been a year since my mom's suicide attempt and my relationship with her had slowly returned to some sort of normalcy (whatever normal was). We had settled into a new rhythm—we spoke on the phone, texted a little, and she checked in with me all the time. She was being a lot more attentive to me than normal, always asking if she could support me in any way. It was new and I felt slightly uncomfortable with the whole thing. *Did I need support?* I wondered. I just needed her to be stable. I needed her to live. On the surface everything looked almost the way it did before her suicide attempt, but deep down I was terrified all the time. I couldn't relax with her. I wanted her to be happy, to want to live, to feel loved—but I didn't trust her anymore. A part of me was wondering if I ever really had. On some level I knew we needed to take a real break. I needed space. I needed to figure out who I was without her, but at the same time the thought of not speaking to her scared me, too. She was the center of my life. Come to think of it, second to Dennis, she was the most important person in my life. Would I be okay without her, even for a while? Would she? I didn't know, but I knew I had to find out. All four of her kids did similar things but in different ways. Since the suicide attempt we'd all distanced ourselves somehow. I was reading a lot about codependency and realized that throughout our lives together, we had leaned on each other in ways that weren't always healthy. Suddenly, after almost thirty years of being a mom, my mother had found herself alone. Returning to Sweden, I sensed something different in her that I couldn't pinpoint, something good, but I still didn't trust her. I didn't think I'd ever be able to trust her again.

In Stockholm we walked the dogs and had long talks. She didn't like the idea of my going to Path of Love. She had been there many years earlier and knew what it was all about. Why was I going? she asked. I didn't have an answer. I didn't really know why I was going. The retreat involved early-life work—going back into childhood, into pain, exploring wounds while using therapy and meditation as a way to heal. I knew it would be intense. Most people who went were experiencing something super challenging in their lives—trauma, divorce, disease, death. At that moment, everything in my life seemed okay. I felt stable. Maybe that was why I was going, I said. Not out of panic, or wanting to fix something that was broken, but to take the next step to becoming a better person.

I spent a beautiful week in Sweden and Mom drove me to the airport for my flight to Germany. We hugged when she dropped me off. "Do you have any idea what you're in for?" she asked. "No," I said, getting out of the car. "But I need this."

When I was booking my stay at the Osho center for the Path of Love retreat, I was obsessive about the lodging. There were so many options, but most were shared rooms or communal living spaces. I wanted my own room. The idea of sharing with a stranger made me uncomfortable. I needed my own space to be. I was told that nothing was available. I begged them to try to accommodate me. At last, one of the facilitators who owned a top-floor apartment at the center where the retreat was being held, offered to rent it to me for cheap.

I landed in Cologne and made my way downtown. A nice woman at the reception desk checked me in and handed me a set of keys. I was early for the retreat and only a few people were around. I lugged my suitcase up five flights and unlocked the door to the apartment where I would be staying. I could hardly believe my luck. It was a penthouse with a huge bedroom and bathroom, and I had my own kitchen. I bounced up and down with excitement.

The rules of the retreat were strict. We were not allowed to communicate with anyone on the outside during our stay and all electronic devices were prohibited. Time between sessions were to be spent in strict silence. I liked to think of myself as a fairly smartphone-balanced person; I used my phone a lot but mostly for work. I wasn't one to have it in my hand at all times. But now, putting it away for a week, I felt like I was about to have my hand chopped off.

Everyone gathered in the main hall for an orientation meeting on the first evening. I was the last person to walk in and the others turned to look at me. I found an empty chair and sat down. The group included forty participants, forty support staff, ten facilitators, and Rafia and Turiya, the founders of the program. I was drawn to Rafia. He was in his sixties, handsome, and very serene looking. "You are in for the ride of your lives," he promised, smiling as he addressed the group. "We are deeply honored to have you here." He looked at me and smiled warmly.

We were each given a big, empty binder and a blank sheet of paper. "The Path of Love has seven keys," Turiya said. "Each key is a doorway to help you go into a deeper space and you will come to understand and embody each of them during the next week. Take out your pens and write this out." She read each key, repeating each one several times. I closed my eyes and let them sink in.

As she read each key of the process out loud, I felt her words begin to move something inside of my chest. One was centered around honesty, and exposing our emotions. Another spoke about how to face our judgments and beliefs. When she read the seventh key out loud, I felt the hairs on the back of my neck stand up. "I will ask for divine help." Turiya repeated it again. "I will ask for divine help." I'd only ever turned to God (or Spirit, or whatever you prefer to call it) for help during moments of despair. I was reminded of my experience during the ayahuasca ceremony years earlier, throwing myself at the floor, praying for relief. Standing in the garden with Pepper when he'd just gone blind, asking Andrea to save him. Clutching my phone to my chest on a beach in Thailand, willing the universe to keep my mother alive. The thought hit me: *I have no relationship with God other than in moments of darkness. I only pray when I'm forced to my knees, close to giving up. What was I hoping to find here?* I still wasn't sure, but knowing that asking for divine help was a part of the process made me feel closer to finding out.

A second sheet of paper was handed out. This one had the rules for the retreat. Rafia explained that the rules were meant to create a strong and deep structure that would support us and our inner search.

Rafia read the rules one at a time. "When not in the group room, you are asked to be in silence," Rafia said. I was expecting this, and understood why. The silence is an important part of the process because it allows us to integrate in between sessions. I'd experienced some of my most life-changing realizations in other retreats as a result of silence. The silence was very, very important, he said.

"No intoxication" was the next rule. It meant we were not to consume any alcohol or nonprescribed drugs during the process. A few people giggled.

"No sexual contact." Rafia didn't explain this rule further. He moved on.

After having listed all the rules for the process, he read the final one. "I agree to follow all the instructions given by the facilitators until the end of the process." Rafia left it at that.

We all signed on the bottom line of the sheet and the assistants collected the papers.

When the session began, we were divided into four groups of nine or ten. Each group will become a kind of family, Rafia said. "You will connect with these people on a level you've never known before. Meet their eyes." I looked around at my group.

There were people of all ages, from all walks of life. Everyone looked nervous.

We were asked to make eye contact with one person in our group and hold that connection. That person would be our partner. A young man I took to be nineteen or twenty met my gaze. He was tall and lean with blue eyes. As I looked at him more closely, he appeared even younger than I'd initially thought. He would be my partner.

We got a moment to familiarize ourselves with each other. My partner's name was Naveen—a sannyasin, or follower of Osho (an Indian mystic also known as Bhagwan Shree Rajnesh). Path of Love and the retreats I'd done prior are rooted in the teachings of Osho, but he is very rarely mentioned. The groups are centered around unconditional love, with no single person to bow to; no one on a pedestal. Naveen was actually my age, about to turn twenty-eight, and had done six or seven groups over the last year. He was a graphic designer and he'd had the same girlfriend for many years. His gaze was piercing and he was intensely dedicated to his spiritual path. I used to put myself in that category. Now I saw myself more as an "easygoing" seeker, if there was such a thing.

When it was my turn to talk, I felt my eyes well up. "My name is Rachel," I said. "I don't know why I'm crying. I live in Aruba. I'm Swedish. I'm married since two years back. I have a good life." As I spoke the last sentence, I choked on my own tears. I felt a sadness so deep it took all of my determination not to break down and sob. I reached for a Kleenex. My life was good. I was in a super-solid place finally. Dennis and I loved each other. We never fought. We were on the same team.

My work fulfilled me. We had money, a beautiful house, and we traveled. Yes, I'd had some crap come up in the past years. But I was over most of it—even with my mom; we had a good relationship again. So why did I have a sinking feeling in my heart? Why did I feel the need to cry? Naveen looked at me with kindness in his eyes.

We returned to our chairs and Rafia and Turiya explained a bit about what the week would entail. We would not see a schedule and would never know in advance what each day had in store. This was to keep us present, to keep our mind from leading us astray.

When the session ended, I returned to my apartment, wrote in my journal, and rolled out my yoga mat. *I don't know why I'm here*, I thought. I just know it's crucial that I am. I sat down on my mat, closed my eyes, and breathed. Suddenly I was jolted backward. I had fallen over. *What just happened?* I wondered. I had fallen asleep sitting up. I didn't even know I was tired. The sky was still bright outside, but I crawled under the covers and fell back asleep.

The next thing I heard was a knock at the door. "Rise and shine!" a voice said. For a moment I didn't know where I was. I reached for my phone for the first time, then remembered I didn't have my phone. I was in Cologne, staying at the Osho center. Today was the first day of Path of Love. "I'm awake," I said to the door. "Good luck today," the voice said. Man. What was I in for? I went into the kitchen. The clock on the wall said 5:35—I had to get going. I changed into yoga pants, a sports bra, and a tank top and brewed myself a cup of tea. It was almost time for the first Dynamic.

The Dynamic Meditation is the "staple" meditation in Osho gatherings and it's designed to get the crazy out—to allow for a release of built-up emotions to make space for what's here, now. It's extremely transformative and also exhausting. The meditation is divided into five stages, each accompanied by very loud music. The first stage is chaotic breathing and it lasts for ten minutes. Focusing only on the exhale, you forcefully breathe out through the nose with the mouth closed while using your entire body to get energy going. The second stage is catharsis—the release. Whatever is inside, you let out. If you are feeling joyful you dance, sing, smile, or laugh. If you feel anger, you scream, punch pillows, curse, or yell. If you feel sad, you cry. It lasts for ten minutes and it's intense. It can be completely overwhelming for first-timers. The third stage is the "Hoo" stage and lasts for ten minutes—you jump up and down, landing on the soles of your feet with your arms stretched up in the air, saying the Sufi chant "*Hoo! Hoo! Hoo!*" The fourth stage is the silent stage and begins when you hear "*Stop!*" At that point, you hold your arms in the air and freeze. When the silent stage is over the celebration begins and you dance. This is the fifth and final stage.

The entire meditation lasts for an hour. The idea is to create a safe space to release all of the emotions we accumulate. Osho, the Indian mystic, believed that the Western mind was too ingrained, too full of worries and problems and tension—we live in the mind. So for us to sit down in silence and expect to be able to meditate is unrealistic. We must first make space for silence to arrive; get into the body and release.

I was nervous about the Dynamic Meditations, even

though I'd done them many times before. I always worried I'd get an asthma attack or wouldn't make it through (which is strange, because physically I'm strong). Something about the Dynamic always triggered within me a fear of not keeping up. I drank my tea and headed downstairs.

When I entered the meditation room, I was handed a blindfold—in Dynamic Meditations everyone wears a blindfold. People were blowing their noses in preparation for the first stage. We were not allowed to bring anything with us, but I snuck my asthma inhaler in my bra. I grabbed a bolster and found a spot in the corner. Even though I rarely used it, knowing my medication was near helped to calm my mind. Everyone in the group was there. When the process was explained, the ones who had never done it looked on with wide eyes. Everyone took their places and a gong sounded, signaling the start of the first stage of meditation. I breathed in through my nose and exhaled forcefully. Snot was coming out of my nose. I wiped my nose on my shirt but didn't stop. The point was for the act to be intense and chaotic enough to oxygenate your entire body, to build up energy. The sound of everyone else breathing kept me going. I couldn't see, but I could sense my surroundings.

After what felt like an eternity, the gong sounded again. The music shifted. Catharsis. Immediately to my left a man let out a primal scream. It was so loud it shocked me. Then everyone was screaming and punching their bolsters. It sounded like we were in a zoo. It was terrifying. "*Fuck! Fuck! Fuck!*" a woman screamed from across the room. The man to my left launched into a complete rage. I knew this was coming—this was what the second stage of a Dynamic was. But it had been years since I'd done it and I felt very small and afraid.

I dropped down to the floor and held up the bolster to defend myself. I was sobbing. I felt so exposed, so unsafe. Madness was going on all around me: people crying, screaming, cursing, stomping their feet, letting out animal noises.

The gong sounded again. It felt like I'd only been there a minute. It was time for the Hoo stage. I was tired and wanted to blow my nose but there was no break in between. I stood and put my arms in the air. Everyone shouted in unison. "*Hoo! Hoo! Hoo!*" I was so exhausted I couldn't keep my arms up straight, so I bent my elbows and kept my hands barely floating above my head. My legs felt like lead. I could barely jump. Finally, someone yelled, "*Stop!*" I froze in place, my arms still up. My heart was pounding and sweat dripped down my face, arms, and legs. I felt like I was in a trance. I lost my sense of space and time. Soon, gentle music filled the room. I swayed from side to side. The music was soft and uplifting and I began to dance.

When the meditation was over and the music stopped, it felt like days had passed. I felt invigorated, energized. It was like the meditation had swept something out of the way and inside I felt empty, but in a good way. I showered, ate breakfast, and still had time for the morning's writing assignment before the next session. There were only two questions.

What really works in your life?

What is missing in your life and what do you feel you need to face in yourself for that to change?

The first question was easy: My relationship with my husband. My dedication to work. Building community, getting things done. Manifesting abundance. My ability to put emotion and pain into words. I left it at that. The second was harder. What was missing in my life that needed to change? "Calm," I wrote. It was a hard pill to swallow and an even harder reality to admit. I am Yoga Girl and calm is missing from my life? I can create moments of serenity and quiet for others, but don't know how to do it for myself. And sex. Our sex life hadn't been the best lately. I'd blamed it on us working together, the stress, the travel, but there was probably more to it, and it was probably me.

When I was finished writing, I walked to the Waiting Room for the second gathering. I chose a chair in the back of the room and sat down. The room filled up quickly. When all the chairs were taken, the assistants closed the door. I looked around. Some people were biting their nails; some were sitting with long spines, eyes closed, seemingly in meditation. Sitting there, I was overcome with exhaustion. Like the previous night on my yoga mat, I kept nodding off. Suppressing a yawn, I wondered, *Why is this called the Waiting Room and what are we waiting for?* I was sure the people around me were asking themselves the same thing.

After what felt like an eternity, the door opened and six people walked in and to the front of the room: a bald man in his fifties; a younger guy with long, curly black hair; a tall, thin woman with hair down to her waist; a lady in her sixties wearing a long, flowy skirt; and a middle-aged man with glasses and a white shirt. In the middle stood a short, beautiful woman who looked to be in her midthirties. She was barefoot and had toe rings and an anklet with tiny little bells that jingled when she moved. "Welcome, everyone," she said, her accent Portuguese. "We are your facilitators. My name is Shubhaa. I am the lead facilitator of group number one." My group. Out of all of them, I was really glad I had Shubhaa. I liked her already.

After the introductions we were guided, one group at a time, into the main hall. The chairs were set up in the same horseshoe formation as the day before, but behind them was a table with ten or so people facing forward. It was super weird. We took our seats. "Welcome to your family," Shubhaa said. "Look around. All of us together will go through some truly transformational things this week. I am here to guide you. In this small group you'll get the chance to stand in front of your group many times and dive into your past, your emotions, your wounds, and have the opportunity to express everything that's moving inside of you now . . . and you'll get to challenge your concepts and beliefs."

I was still so tired I could barely follow her words—I could barely keep my eyes open. I worried that I wouldn't be able to hold my head up much longer. It was as if the moment this process began I started deflating. I just wanted to sleep.

Shubhaa continued. "The topic of this first exercise is this: How are you feeling right now—and what do you truly long for in your life?" The group was silent. I was terrified. *Don't pick me*, I prayed silently.

"Who would like to be the first person to stand up?" she asked. For a long time, no one moved. Finally, the tall guy sitting across from me stood. He towered over everyone. He was handsome, probably in his forties, athletic with blond, thinning hair and dark circles under his eyes. "Hi, everyone," he said. "My name is Bas, and I'm feeling good. What do I long for? I don't know. I work a high-powered job. I'm a little bit tired, maybe." I didn't believe him. "I don't know why I'm here," he said. "I met a girl. She recommended it. I run a big company. I have two hundred employees. And I work all the time. But I like my work. Everything is good." He looked at Shubhaa, for a cue to continue. She said nothing. "That's it, I guess?" Shubhaa smiled at him. "Thank you, Bas. Who's next?"

The woman next to me stood up. She was short, with curly red hair and round hips. "My name is Tatiana," she said, speaking with a heavy Finnish accent. "I'm from Helsinki. I am feeling nervous about being here. I am a single mother. My daughter is sixteen. She worries about me." "Why does she worry about you?" Shubhaa asked. "I haven't been very happy." Tatiana said. "My mother passed away last year." Her face was etched with pain. "She was my everything, my mother," she said. "But there hasn't been any time for grieving. I have a business and my daughter and I am very busy." "And what do you long for, Tatiana?" Shubhaa asked. "Happiness," Tatiana said. "Joy. I haven't felt joyful in a long time." Her eyes filled with tears as she sat down.

The next person was a dark-haired woman. She may have been in her late thirties or she might have been older. She was wearing heavy eye makeup and her forehead was as smooth as ice. She looked angry, even when she smiled. "My name is Bianca," she said. "I am from France but I live in Florida with my husband and my son. Or, I guess it's just me and my son now. We have a beautiful home there. It's right on the ocean. I'm an interior designer." "And how are you feeling, Bianca?" Shubhaa asked. "I don't know," the woman replied. "I have a few reasons to be here, I guess. My husband cheated on me. Now we are divorcing but he wants to take my business and the house and everything I own. It's very unfair. I guess I'm a little angry." Shubhaa asked, "What do you long for, Bianca?" Bianca was silent for a long time. "I don't want to feel this way," she said finally. "This is not me, the way I am feeling. I'm so angry. I want to be happy."

I panicked every time someone finished. I didn't want to be next. I was so tired I could barely keep my eyes open. Naveen stood. "Hi, guys. I'm from Germany. I'm really excited to be here," he said. *Excited?* I thought to myself. *What a cocky guy. It's clear everyone here is going through something, everyone is sad, tired, overworked, angry, and this guy is excited?* I didn't believe him either. "This is my sixth Osho group in a year," he said. "It came highly recommended. I long to deepen my connection with God, with the universe. I want to deepen my meditation practice."

A woman in her forties, beautiful with a round face, brown eyes, and dark hair down past her shoulders, looked at each of us. "My name is Devika," she said, trying not to cry. "I'm a mother of three beautiful boys and I don't know why I'm here. I love my husband. My boys. My life. Everything is good. I just feel like I've lost something. Like I've lost a bit of myself . . . I think I long for alone time. I want to remember what it's like to be me again. I don't want to be just a mother, just a wife. I want to find myself." When Devika sat down, I knew I should have stood, to get it over with, but I put my hands to my face and realized I was crying. Using the sleeve of my sweater, I wiped away my tears. *I can't stand*, I thought. *I'm too tired.*

Two more men stood. The first, Peter, said he was confused and searching for wisdom. "I want to be in the know," he said. "I want clarity. I want to know why we are all here. The meaning of life. I contemplate it often." When he sat down, the last man in the group stood up. He was handsome, with dark brown eyes and a bit of stubble across a tan face. Mala beads were dangling around his neck. "My name is Matteo. I'm from Chile. I was excited to be here but now I am very nervous. I've been struggling with some anger issues. Some family traumas. Things I want to resolve. I feel like there is some serious darkness inside me. Troubles from my childhood. I had a very challenging childhood and I think it still lives in me." Matteo said he longed for peace of mind. "I just want peace."

And then it was just two of us left. Another girl and me. I couldn't move. The other girl stood. She was thin, with blond hair and big glasses sitting on the tip of her nose. "My name is Anna," she said. "I'm from Switzerland. I just went through a breakup. My boyfriend left me, with no warning. Everyone leaves me. I don't know what I'm doing wrong." She wiped her eyes with a Kleenex. "I long for love," she said. "Real, true love. I don't have anyone." She burst into tears. Shubhaa walked up to her and placed a hand on her shoulder. "You are very brave, coming here. Very strong," she said. Her words seemed to calm Anna and she sat down.

I was the only one left. I wanted to stand but I felt like I had melted into the chair. After a long moment, Shubhaa asked, "Rachel? Would you like to stand up?" I didn't, but even more I wanted everyone to stop looking at me. The moment I stood and looked out at the group I burst into tears. I just stood there, in front of everyone, crying. I felt so embarrassed. "Can I touch your arm?" Shubhaa asked. I nodded, and she placed both hands on my upper arms and stroked them. I was calmed by her touch. "How are you feeling, Rachel?" she asked. I tried to speak, but the tears started to flow again. "I'm just so . . . tired," I cried. It was true. I'd never been so tired. It was as if the speed of my life and all the pain I'd felt over the last two years were hitting me all at once. "And what do you long for, Rachel?" Shubhaa asked. "I want to sleep," I said, smiling a little. "I just want to rest." Shubhaa smiled at me. "Thank you, Rachel."

I was emotionally overwrought, everyone was, but the day was just beginning. We were about to start the next exercise— about how we were perceived by people who knew little or nothing about us. Every person was to stand in front of the group and receive feedback from other participants. "We want honest, raw truth," Shubhaa said.

Tatiana started us off. "Anna, what do you think of me?" Following Shubhaa's instructions, Anna responded, "Tatiana, I see you as someone who is a very kind person. A good friend." Shubhaa interrupted her. "Thank you, Anna, but that's not what we are looking for here. Of course Tatiana has many beautiful and amazing qualities, but what this exercise is about is looking at the shadow side. If you look at Tatiana right now, what do you see? What is the real truth?" Anna looked at Tatiana for a long time. "I understand. Tatiana . . . I see you as someone who has had a very hard life." "Thank you, Anna," said Shubhaa. "Tatiana, please continue."

"Bas, what do you think of me?"

"Tatiana, I see you . . . as a little bit standoffish," he said.

"Naveen, what do you think of me?"

"Tatiana, I see you as someone who has had a lot of struggle in their past," he said.

"Rachel, what do you think of me?" she asked.

I didn't want to hurt her feelings, but I wanted to be truthful. She did look like someone who had had a very hard life. Wrinkles were carved into her face and her forehead was lined from frowning. Her arms were crossed over her chest. "Tatiana, I see you as someone who is fighting upstream," I said.

When everyone answered, Tatiana looked visibly upset. "I didn't think you would answer me like this," she said. "It's all true. I mean, yes, I have had a very tough life. But I see myself as a very happy person. I don't want to be seen as someone who has had a hard life. I am so much more than that."

I had never looked at anyone with such unfiltered honesty. My heart pounded when it was my turn to stand up in front of the group. I tried to think loving thoughts—I hoped they saw me as a nice person. Their answers shocked me. "Rachel, I see you as someone who has a wall up," Anna said. "Rachel, I see you as someone who is a control freak," said Matteo. "I see you as someone who has a deep, deep sadness inside," Devika said. "I see you as someone who deep down believes she is ugly," Bas said. "I see you as a perfectionist," Peter said. "I see you as someone who is very angry, deep within," Tatiana said.

Naveen was the last one. "I see you as someone who carries the weight of the world on her shoulders," he said.

I just stood there. "How does this make you feel?" Shubhaa asked. "Sad," I said, starting to cry. "Really, really sad. I don't feel like I am that person they're talking about. Or maybe I am, but I don't want it to show."

"And what happens if you would show the world your true colors?" Shubhaa asked. "No one would want to be with me," I said.

Was that really who I was? Controlling? Sad? A perfection-ist? Shubhaa called what we were doing "shadow work." It was deeply transformative, she said. The Path of Love process was not just about finding our way to love and light, but about looking at our shadow side, our dark side, and, instead of sup-pressing those parts of us, giving them space and letting them show. "When we stop hiding these sides of ourselves, we can transform them into something beautiful," she said. "This pro-cess is about welcoming every part of who you are."

We were later asked to write a letter stating our commitment to ourselves. "I commit to letting myself be vulnerable, seen, and held," I wrote. I wondered how in the hell I was going to make it through the rest of the week. It had only been a few hours and already I felt like I had learned so much about myself, but it didn't change the exhaustion and deep sense of sadness I felt.

When it was time to go back into session, I noticed the chairs were set up differently. They were grouped in pairs, facing each other. Matteo ended up sitting across from me. The question we were instructed to ask each other was "At the end of your life, will you be able to look back and feel content about the life you have lived?"

Matteo went first. "I'm so angry," he said. "I don't want to die knowing I spent most of my life holding on to anger and resentment."

When it was my turn, I spoke with confidence. "If I would die today, I would feel like I did my best," I said. "At least I hope so. I have loved. I love. A lot. I've seen the world. But, also, I have spent too many nights on the couch watching TV. I could be taking better care of my body. I could be having more sex with my husband. He loves me so much. Also, I think there is a lot of healing left for me to do." I was surprised at how easy it was to share intimate pieces of my life and my relationships with a complete stranger.

When the sharing part was over, we were divided into two long lines and told to hold the gaze of the person across from us. My person was a redheaded woman with piercing green eyes and freckles. I didn't know her name, and holding her gaze felt awkward and uncomfortable. Every few minutes, we were instructed to take another step toward each other. Why was it so hard to look her in the eye? I asked myself. I taught yoga for a living. I guided people toward intimacy and connection. Why was this so hard?

Rafia guided us until our foreheads were touching. I was relieved because I couldn't see her eyes anymore. The connection felt nice. At the end, we embraced. I felt uncomfortable again. The music changed. People started to move around the room.

I went to a corner to hide. Shubhaa called me out. "Rachel, let's go!" I shook my head. "Come on," she urged. "There is a child inside you. She wants to come out and play. It's been a heavy day. Dance!" She took my hand and pulled me toward the middle of the room. I felt like I was in school and everyone was going to laugh at me. I waved my arms and spun myself around. "You did good," Shubhaa whispered. "Little bits at a time."

Finally we got a break for tea and snacks. "Rest for a little and get your energy back," Rafia said. "You are going to need it." We were instructed to return in forty-five minutes with a full bottle of water and a towel. I arrived early. Once everyone was back, Rafia gave us our next task. "You are about to go into a strong group meditation," he said. "The hall upstairs has been transformed to a safe, sacred space for you to burn through your emotions. It's a place to feel your feelings and to let old emotions come up, catch fire and burn. It will bring you tremendous relief. There are mattresses and pillows and blankets laid out across the room. Find a mattress, make it yours, and go into whatever emotion is there. There are people there to support you and keep you safe. Use your towel to twist, cry into, punch, and cover yourself. Go deep. Your longing is burning in your heart and it wants to lead you home. Follow your group leader into the room, holding your partner's hand."

The air was electric. I found Naveen and we followed our group upstairs to the main hall. The room had been transformed. The lights were turned low and mattresses with pillows and blankets covered the floor. Music blared. I chose a mattress in the corner. The doors closed and Rafia spoke on a microphone, guiding us to our breath, into our bodies. Clutching my pillow, I closed my eyes. I could feel the beating of my heart. I covered my face with the towel and cried into it.

Rafia guided us deeper, drawing on real-life examples of pain. He spoke of loss, struggle, and heartache. Soon, everyone was crying. The music intensified. People around me transitioned from sadness and tears to anger. I heard people screaming, punching pillows, and banging their fists into their mattresses. Someone near me had flown into a rage. "*Fuck you you motherfucking cunt fuck!*" he shouted. I recognized the voice as Matteo's and opened my eyes to a terrifying scene. Three assistants were holding him back while he kicked a bolster that was held by another assistant. The assistants taunted him. "Is that all you've got? Huh?" I watched as Matteo's eyes went dark. It wasn't him anymore, only his rage. He fought and fought until he finally collapsed on the floor, sobbing. The assistants surrounded him, holding him and stroking his back and his head. As I watched the scene play out, my rational mind thought, *This is genius*. I actually saw the release of emotion right in front of me—the healing. *It's fucking insane that we hold this inside*, I thought. That this exists within us. Letting it out isn't what's crazy—holding it in is.

I wanted to feel angry, too. I was on the outside looking in instead of going into my own experience. I tried punching my pillow, but I was too tired, and it felt like too much effort. I felt like I couldn't move. Someone squatted down beside me. I didn't recognize the voice. "Do it anyway," he said. "Punch it anyway. Even if you're not angry. Even if you feel nothing. Let the body lead. Just punch it."

I did as I was told. I punched the pillow. Again and again and again. I felt my anger rise to the surface. I was angry to be there. *Why am I in this room full of crazy people?* I wondered. *I don't belong here.* Or maybe I did. Maybe it was all the external bullshit—the things I'd learned in the outside world that made me feel like I didn't belong. I punched the pillow again and I felt anger rising within me. *Why was I here? Why did I have to go and do crazy things like punch pillows in a dark room full of angry people when I could be at home with my husband in peace? Why did life bring me so many struggles?* I started yelling, angry at the world, and roared and punched until I crumpled in tears onto my mattress. I saw Pepper in front of me. I was hugging the pillow but I was also hugging him. Pepper. My baby. I missed him so much. I couldn't breathe. I heard Shubhaa's voice. "Can we hold you?" she asked. While she held me, someone else placed their hands on my feet and squeezed them. "Why are you sad?" Shubhaa asked. "Tell me." I could barely get the words out. "He . . . he died. Pepper. He died. I should have saved him, but I didn't. It was my fault. Pepper, my dog, I loved him so much." Shubhaa held her face against mine. I wondered if she was surprised that Pepper was a dog. Was it strange that I was feeling so much sadness over a pet? "Wow," she said. "Look at all the love you have for him. There is so much love. Can you feel it?" I nodded yes. "Just stay with that for a moment," she said. "Stay with the love. You have so much love for him. That's why the pain is big, because the love was big. Don't leave it—stay, right there. Just feel." I stopped crying and sat in stillness. I felt the love. It was enveloped in a big layer of sadness, but the love was there. Oceans of it. For Pepper.

"Can I ask you a question?" Shubhaa said. Again I nodded. "If you could have saved him, would you have?" Her question stunned me. I would have given anything—done anything to save Pepper. "Of course," I said. "But you couldn't," she said.

I don't know what it was about that simple sentence—whether it was the release of anger and pain and sadness I'd buried, or all the emotions I had from the intensity of the retreat—but it changed everything for me. "You couldn't." It was true. I couldn't save him. If I could have, I would have. But I couldn't. Life didn't work that way. "If I could have saved him, I would have," I repeated. "And what does that tell you?" Shubhaa asked. "Maybe . . ." I said. "Maybe it wasn't my fault."

Hearing myself say the words, I felt a heavy weight lift from my chest. Pepper's death wasn't my fault. I loved him more than anything. If I could have saved him, I would have. I couldn't and he died. It wasn't my fault. I exhaled and fell fast asleep. Right there on my mattress, with people all around me, I slept. It was as if releasing the guilt I'd held on to surrounding Pepper's death had pulled some kind of plug. It wasn't my fault. My entire body let go.

That night, after dinner and meditation, I returned to my room for bed. As I went to close the blinds, I glanced across the courtyard to a light in a window on the other side. I could see a woman sitting there, looking out at the night, breastfeeding her baby. I felt a sudden yearning in the bottom of my belly. They looked so peaceful. An unexpected thought came my way. *I want that.* I closed the blinds and went to sleep.

On the third day, I left my inhaler behind. I had gained trust in the group. I felt safer than I had when I got there, even though

I suspected the sessions would intensify. I trusted a little more. Shubhaa started off with a question that related to my epiphany about Pepper the day before. "Why had I felt responsible for Pepper, for his life and his death? Where did the guilt stem from?" She didn't say anything more than that. That was how things went in sessions with Shubhaa—she didn't interrogate us, or ask a bunch of questions leading up to what she wanted to know. She just threw it out there.

What was the root of my guilt? I knew the answer to the question but it stuck in the back of my throat, like I was about to vomit. Something wanted out, but I was having a hard time purging it. "I think it's related to my mom," I said after a few minutes of silence. Shubhaa didn't speak, which prompted me to fill in the silence. "She has tried to commit suicide several times. It happened last year again. I was the one who saved her. Since I was little, I've felt like I was the one responsible for her life."

I spoke calmly, almost matter-of-factly. I knew I was speaking from my logical mind. *Yes, this happened. Yes, it sucks. But I'm over it. Right?* "What's happening in your body now?" Shubhaa asked. "Close your eyes. Feel this in your body. Say that sentence again. 'I feel like I'm responsible for my mother's life.'" Taking a deep breath, I began to speak. "I feel . . . I feel . . ." I was choking on my words. "I feel like I'm responsible for my mother's life." My throat closed and I couldn't catch my breath. I grabbed my throat and gasped. Shubhaa ran toward me and waved for the assistants to follow her. She rubbed my back. "You are safe here," she said, trying to soothe me. "It's safe here. It's safe to be in your own body. You are safe." I began to gag.

The responsibility was choking me. "Basket!" Shubhaa yelled. I vomited into the basket but nothing came out. "You were just a child," Shubhaa said. I clung to her words. *I was just a child. It wasn't my fault that she wanted to die.* I felt myself calm down. I was awestruck by how much was moving inside of me. The session ended and when I left to return to my apartment, I still felt like there was something festering in my body—something that needed to come out.

That afternoon, we had another intense meditation. I tried getting angry, but instead I just sat on my mattress, crying, thinking about Andrea. I wondered if I would ever be done processing her death. I wanted her to come to me in a vision like Pepper did the day before, but I didn't see her. I just felt the pain.

At the end of the day we had satsang—a sacred gathering. It felt like Savasana at the end of a yoga class. Calming. Beautiful. Back in my apartment, uneasiness set in. I felt alone and panicky. *Why hadn't I stayed in a dorm or communal hall, or at least had a roommate?* Instead, it was just me in that big apartment I'd fought so hard to get.

I showered, trying to wash the panic away. I brewed a cup of tea and sat in silence, attempting to meditate. I tried all of my methods—rolling out my yoga mat, burning palo santo, journaling. Nothing made it subside. I didn't even know where it was coming from.

I went to bed, hoping it would go away. As soon as I tried to sleep, the anxiety took over completely. My throat closed and I couldn't get a breath. I began to panic the way I did when I was attacked by the dogs in my street the year before—I just couldn't breathe anymore. I wanted to call Rose, or Dennis, but I couldn't. Gasping for air I was certain I was about to die and there was no one to help me. The center was closed and I was alone. *I'm going to die here and no one knows.*

On some level I understood that what was happening was a panic attack, but I had also convinced myself I was dying. I opened the wardrobe doors, pulled out my suitcase, and dug out my computer. As I waited for it to turn on, my breath was barely present. Black spots flickered in front of my face. I felt my chest tightening. I opened up Skype and dialed the emergency number on the welcome sheet. It was the middle of the night. A woman answered, her voice tired. "Osho UTA, can I offer my assistance?" "I'm dying," I said. "I'm dying. Help. I'm dying. Please—I can't breathe. I'm on the top floor. I'm alone. My name is Rachel. Please help." The woman's voice was calm. Too calm. "We will send someone right away, stay on the line with me," she said. "Deep breaths. Can you explain to me what is happening right now? What's going on in your body?"

I realized everyone on the staff was trained in managing trauma and panic. The woman knew what to say. By the time someone knocked on my door I had calmed down a little. I was embarrassed. *I should have dealt with this on my own*, I thought.

When I opened the door, Shubhaa and Turiya were standing there. I burst into tears. They sat me down and Shubhaa rubbed my back. "Explain to us what happened," Turiya said. She was the creator of the process—the teacher of teachers. I looked for words, but what spilled out were words I hadn't realized were there. "My mom did Path of Love," I said. "And then she did the therapist training with you last year. And in the middle of it she tried to commit suicide. You couldn't help her, and you let her go out into the world to help other people when she is the one who needs help. I don't trust you. I don't trust any of this." I was completely stunned by what came out of my mouth. I didn't even know I had those feelings. They must have been buried deep.

Turiya spoke first. "Trust is the most fundamental component of this process," she said. "Without it, you are just out at sea on your own. Trust is your buoy. It's how we navigate through these difficult waters together. It is not strange that these feelings have surfaced. You are very brave for sharing them with us."

She went on to tell me about my mother's training. "She did not tell us she had tried to commit suicide—we didn't know," she said. "It came out in the middle of an intimate circle; she hadn't notified me in advance. We took it very seriously. Suicide is a very, very serious thing. Had we known she was suicidal prior to applying, she would never have been accepted to the program. But there we were, in the midst of it. Sometimes life happens that way. You do the best you can with the cards you are dealt. We did, your mother did. As are you, right now." This was all news to me. "I am so worried about her," I said. "And now she is out there trying to help people. And it terrifies me. And I thought, what if she became this way because of the training? Not only did you not help her, but she became even worse."

Turiya put a hand on my shoulder. "You and your mother are on very different paths," she said. "For some, awakening is a slower process. It is important that you distinguish your process from your mother's. And I ask you to trust us. You are supported here. You are held. Your mother's path is hers, not yours."

"That's what happened today in the group session," I said. "I just touched a little sliver of the reality of her suicide attempt and I had to vomit. It's like it's stuck in my body. I don't feel safe anywhere."

"Just the fact that you are here, now, asking for help, is a huge step," Shubhaa said. "This pain is real, the fear is real. It sits in your body. But it's also old. It's not playing out in the here and now. You need to rid yourself of the old, close the wound, and manifest a life where you are independent of it. Where you know, deeply, that your mother's life doesn't lie in your hands. What a weight to carry! Aren't you tired?"

I started to cry. "Exhausted," I said.

"Are you okay to sleep on your own? We can have one of the assistants sleep in here with you if you'd like."

"I'm alright," I said. "I trust the process." As I said it, I knew it was true. I trusted the process. I was grateful for them.

I went back to bed and said a prayer.

Dear Universe,

Please help me face this pain so I can heal it. I don't want it to dictate my life anymore. Please help me get through this and help keep me as one, whole person.

For the first time I felt like I could speak the truth without blame or resentment. I had spent my life holding my mother's pain. I had to put half the earth between us for me to find my own way—for me to find myself. When I was with her, I had to dull my shine because I felt like there was never enough for her. I made myself small when actually I was a bright, shining star. Who gave her the right to be @yoga_mum on Instagram? Yoga, Yoga Girl—that was my identity. She didn't even do yoga! It was crazy, really. I couldn't spend the rest of my life weighed down by my fear of her taking her own life. I had to start living for me.

I went to the next meditation with the overwhelming need to have my own space. Standing in the middle of the room, I stretched my arms straight out, palms up, as if to say, "Stop!" I envisioned a force field around me, my subtle energy setting a strong but gentle boundary for myself. No one could cross it unless I allowed them to. I visualized my mother on the other side and me, speaking loudly, telling her, "No! No, you can't be 'Yoga mom.' No, you can't go everywhere I go. No, you can't make your children my responsibility. No, no, no!"

Leaving the room, I felt strong and whole. "You're glowing—like a star," Shubhaa whispered. "Like a star." I felt like a star. Like I was shining.

Toward the end of the retreat we did something called a Peace Walk. The idea was to walk until we were able to clearly state our longing to the universe. Everyone around me had epiphanies. I walked and walked but nothing came. *Maybe I'd had all of my epiphanies earlier in the week*, I thought. How many realizations about life can a person have in such a short time? I continued walking, but something wasn't right. I felt heavy and tired again.

I realized that Rafia was walking alongside me. He took my hand. "You have to put her down," he said. I knew who he meant. I was still carrying the weight of my mother. "She's small, but she's heavy," he said. "I can't put her down," I said. Tears sprang to my eyes. "If I do, she . . . she . . ." "She, what?" Rafia asked. "She might die." Saying it out loud was terrifying. "It must be exhausting, feeling responsible for her," Rafia said. "And you do it out of love, of course. But are you really helping her?"

I didn't know what he meant. "You love her so much—you want her to stay alive," he said. "To live a long life. But sometimes, if we've never been on our own two feet, we don't know that we are capable to deal with life ourselves." *Is that what I've done? By holding her and worrying and caring for the whole family and being the fixer and the rescuer?*

We continued to walk. "She is in charge of her own life," Rafia said. "Don't take her power away—don't trick yourself into thinking you can take her power away. What she does with her life is her business. Not yours."

Anger bubbled up in my throat. "She doesn't know how to care for herself," I said. "If it wasn't for me, she would be dead."

Rafia stopped and looked at me. "Who made you God?" I looked into his eyes. His eyes were serious, and warm. "What's the worst thing that could happen if you just put her down?" he asked. I closed my eyes. I knew the answer. "She could die," I said. Rafia's eyes were piercing mine. "So. Let her die then," he said. *Let her die?* I couldn't speak. "It's her life," Rafia said. "It's her decision. You are not God—you don't decide who lives and who dies. You can try, but it's not going to give you anything other than exhaustion and pain. Let her go. Let her live her own life. Trust that she can care for herself. Let her live. Or let her die. Let her be." He squeezed my hand and left my side.

I kept walking. Let her die? Another truth. I knew he was right. If letting her go meant letting her die, then that's what I had to do. It was a hard, hard pill to swallow. My mother was too heavy to carry. That's why I was so tired. I couldn't carry her anymore. I had to put her down. I had to let her go. I dropped to my knees.

> *Dear God,*
> *Please take the burden that is my mother off my shoulders. I can't carry her anymore. Please keep her safe. Keep her whole. Please help her find her own light. I am letting go now. Amen.*

I don't normally like the term *God*—I always say Spirit, or Universe, or Love. But God sounded right in my prayer. I need space, God. From her. I can't keep her in my life. Not right now. Wherever this process leads me, I need to get there on my own. I need to find out what it's like to live just for me. I feel clear and calm about this decision. I have let go. I am done.

I felt a presence of warmth fill my heart. Andrea. She was here. I'd longed for her. I saw her in front of me, laughing, shining, and I realized: everything I ever wanted to be I saw in her. She was so very much herself—she was all the sweet juiciness I always longed for in myself. She had all the shine I never felt I was worthy of. Being with her brought out the most beautiful version of me. She never needed a Path of Love—she lived it. That's part of why I missed her so much: because being with her reminded me of something I always felt was missing. By shining her light I felt I had permission to do the same. I missed her so much. The warmth around my heart intensified. I reminded myself: *the pain is big because the love was big.*

I walked out of Path of Love after eight days of the most intense, heart-opening healing I had ever experienced and I was very clear about what I had to do. I needed to separate from my mom at least for a while. I didn't know what it meant, or how long it would last. I just knew I needed space.

When I turned on my phone for the first time and went to social media, the first thing that popped up was a post from her. While I was away she had changed her Instagram name— she was no longer @yoga_mum. I couldn't believe it. All on her own—I hadn't had contact with anyone.

My mom had sent me many messages while I was away. It took me two days to work up the courage to call. When we finally spoke, she sounded nervous, like she knew what was coming.

"Why did you change your Instagram name?" I asked.

"I don't know, I just had this strange realization . . . Was it strange that I tried to be yoga mom? I mean, yoga is your thing. You are Yoga Girl. I don't even like yoga! I don't know why I did that. I'm sorry."

My heart softened. While I was away working on myself, she had been doing some work, too.

I explained that I needed space, and for us not to be in contact for a while. I could tell I was breaking her heart, but it had to be done. I was doing this for me. "I don't know how long it will be," I said. "I just need space to figure myself out, and I can't do it together with you."

I think on some level she understood. It wasn't about her personally—it was about our past together and the heavy energy that sat there. It was about my wounds, my journey, and the changes I had to make for me. Although we'd struggled so much in our past, there was so much love there. I didn't want our challenges to overcloud the love that had always been so present between us. She had done her absolute best. I loved her deeply. But finally, for the first time in my life, I loved myself more.

21

THE BEGINNING

Seeing Dennis's face when I returned home from Path of Love was the most beautiful thing. My soul mate. My love. I told him everything I'd learned. Things I'd never told him before, things I'd been ashamed of, my mistakes, my struggles. I shared it all. We cried together and afterward drove to a secluded beach on the north shore. We made love there and then I lay with my head on his chest, listening to his heartbeat, tears streaming down my cheeks. "What's wrong?" he asked. "I'm just so happy." It was true. I had so much to be grateful for. My life was so full. For the first time in my life, I felt completely whole.

I woke up in the middle of the night two weeks later with my breasts aching. I didn't have to count back the days to know that I'd gotten pregnant that afternoon on the beach. I didn't have to look back over my life to know the healing that had to take place for that moment to happen.

Dennis and I were overjoyed. I thought I would be terrified, but I wasn't. I felt ready. Everything was so serendipitous. So perfect. I knew it was a girl.

We decided to name her Lea, the name I'd dreamed of for my daughter since I was a little girl. In the Bible, Lea and Rachel were sisters. I always wanted a sister when I was little, someone to share secrets with and whisper under the covers to at night. Dennis loved the name, but if we had a boy? he wondered. I didn't need to wait for the ultrasound—I knew it was a girl.

From the moment I found out I was pregnant I was convinced the baby would be born on the day of Andrea's passing. I did the math in my head—we conceived in the beginning of June, so nine months ahead . . . The date would fall somewhere at the end of February or the beginning of March. Andrea died March 10. Something inside of me just clicked when I made the connection; I felt absolutely relieved. It made total sense! Of course the baby would be born then! The midwives gave me a due date of February 28 and told me "babies come in their own time," and that going so far overdue was rare and highly unusual and to not get my head too wrapped around a specific day. I didn't listen to them—they didn't know the pain and the miracles I'd seen over the past three years. They didn't know Andrea, they didn't know us. But I knew: March 10 was the date. Finally, the darkest day of my life would be transformed into something light. Death would become birth. All was happening in divine order.

The pregnancy started off with some nausea, but after that everything came easy. I started feeling a reverence for my body that I'd never experienced before. I always had a deep connection to my body and felt both strong and flexible thanks to a decade of intense yoga practice; I could handstand with ease and while flowing from pose to pose on the mat I'd have moments when I felt like I was flying—I loved, loved my body. But being pregnant brought on an entirely different kind of appreciation. I couldn't just "do" things—tricky arm balances, dance, run, hug—I could create life. Me! Creating a human being! The thought was mind-boggling. I started gaining weight and it was wonderful. I understood what people meant when they spoke about "pregnancy glow"—it's not just the beauty of creating life but the inner glow that comes from taking part in something so sacred and so ancient it connects us to the dawn of time. I was nauseous and dizzy and my boobs hurt, but I'd never felt more beautiful. I remembered the cacao shaman's words to me from many years before: "When you have a daughter, she won't carry any past pain with her in life. The pain your family has suffered for generations ends with you." When you have a daughter. A daughter. Dennis wasn't convinced (he thought maybe we'd have a boy), and we hadn't even had the gender-revealing ultrasound yet. But I knew. A part of me wished for the baby to carry some of Andrea's spirit with her. "What if the baby is Andrea, coming back to us?" I asked Dennis one day early in the pregnancy. He didn't like the sound of that. "No," he said. "That's not how this works. Maybe you can talk to Andrea through the baby, but the baby is her own little being." I accepted it, but secretly hoped meeting the baby would be like meeting my best friend again. It wasn't until I got further along in the pregnancy and began truly tapping into the spirit growing inside of me that I understood that Dennis was right.

This little girl was entirely her own little person—of course she was! I could already feel her personality, her heart, her soul. She was feisty, strong, stubborn—a lot like me—and also calm, sweet, patient . . . a lot like Dennis. This wasn't the reincarnation of Andrea, however beautiful (and slightly insane) that thought was. This baby was, well, Poppy. We'd started calling her our little poppy seed, since that was the size she was when we found out we were pregnant. The name stuck, and for the remainder of the pregnancy we called her Poppy.

A few months later, my mom came to Aruba to visit. She'd booked the tickets before I went to Path of Love and asked if it was still okay to come. Yes, I said, but she had to find her own place to stay. I wondered if I was being harsh. We hadn't spoken for months. I hadn't told her about the baby. We didn't tell anyone. It was too early; she was still our secret.

Mom arrived with Maia and I went to see them. I wanted to see how I felt. A part of me missed my mother deeply. I missed laughing with her, but I wasn't ready to go back to what was before.

She seemed happy and calm. She told me she'd joined AA. "I'm sober now," she said. That took me by surprise. She drank, sure, but I never saw her as an alcoholic. "I had a wake-up call," she said. "It was the day after you finished Path of Love and you still hadn't called me," she said. "I knew since you didn't call me right away, that you had had realizations that were going to lead you away from me. It was so painful. I drank a lot that night, went out with my girlfriends, and in the middle of the night I was awoken by the sound of a loud voice. 'Enough,' it said. 'You need to be fully present now. Enough.' That day, I went to my first meeting." I did the math in my head. *That was the same day we conceived the baby. Could it be . . . ?*

My thoughts were interrupted by my sister. "Let's swim," she said. Maia looked healthy. Normally, I would have peppered her with questions about her life and Mom's, then offered to help with whatever was happening, but I didn't. Maia was my sister, not my daughter. I loved her and cared for her, but I wasn't going to allow anything to become my burden. We swam, then floated for a while, looking at the sky. "Things are actually really good at home," Maia told me. "Something has shifted. There is something about AA. I think it's doing something. She is different. Calmer." I smiled. "That's good," I said. I wanted my mother to be well. If AA was the way, I supported it. Just then, my mother walked out into the water. "Can I join you?" she asked. She looked so little, but so grown-up. *I wonder if she knows I've let her go*, I thought. "I'm pregnant," I said instead. "You're what?" "I'm pregnant." My mom looked at me. Maia took my hand. All three of us started to cry. My mother hugged me tightly. Feeling her arms around me, I exhaled with relief. Somehow I knew then, there: everything was going to be okay.

Things settled into a new normal after that. I didn't feel the need to separate myself from her anymore, and I didn't feel tense when we spent time together. I felt free. It was like the baby brought about a new level of connection in our relationship—now we got to love someone we were both a part of, instead of being so intently focused on each other. I started having regular contact with my mom again, but in a way that didn't feel suffocating. She continued with AA and I had learned to draw the line between her life and mine. Stepping into the journey of becoming a mother brought about a new sense of respect and reverence for my mom. She had done this four times—all alone. She'd been through hell and back and had managed to raise four beautiful kids. I hadn't even given birth yet, and I was already feeling overwhelmed with what was ahead. I was humbled and gained a new respect for everything my mother had been through to bring me and my siblings into the world. A part of me was terrified; *Would I manage? Was I ready?* I knew I could only do my best, just like my mom had. When I was three months pregnant someone told me something that would forever change the way I looked at my past. When we are pregnant with a daughter, we actually carry two generations in our womb. The eggs that will one day become my daughter's children are already inside of her, meaning they are inside of me. This means that when my mother was pregnant with me, she also had our little poppy seed inside of her. The three of us have been intertwined since before I was born. What if all of this was fated? What if we were meant to go through life just like this, for this moment to arrive? What if we'd been waiting for Poppy all along?

In August I announced my pregnancy on social media. Sharing my pregnancy with the world felt so special—I'd shared everything with my community over the past few years and taking them along on such a happy journey felt like solidifying a new chapter. For the most part, everything went as expected. I continued with work and travel and we prepared for Island Yoga to open at the beginning of the New Year. Dennis was so excited to be a dad. We went to our second ultrasound and found out that, indeed, it was a girl. I was overjoyed. Every morning I would roll out my yoga mat, sit down, put my hands on my belly, and talk to her. I'd talk about how excited I was to meet her and tell her everything I'd been through and all the things it took for us to be there. I'd tell her about all the beauty of life and the things I loved and struggled with. I'd tell her about Andrea, about how much I missed her. "Tell her I love her, okay?" I'd ask. "Tell her we missed her at the wedding and that it was beautiful. Tell her Pepper peed on my dress—she would have fallen over laughing, I know it. Tell her we hung her bridesmaid's dress in a corner and lit a candle and made an altar and everyone went to sit there. Tell her I miss her, all the time." I'd practice yoga and move and stretch and breathe and in the end, I'd sit in meditation. It was like having her inside of me intensified my ability to sit in silence, to be present, to feel. "Look," I'd whisper. "The sun is rising." And we'd sit there, watching the sun rise. Pregnancy was so beautiful. It was like the puzzle pieces I had spent my life trying to figure out all fell into place. In a way, it felt as if everything was meant to happen the way it did, in the time it did, so I could watch my belly grow and feel everything connect in time for her to be born.

When I got into my third trimester, things started getting challenging. My belly was huge—really huge—and already from week thirty-six the midwives started telling me to get ready for an early labor. "This is already a big baby!" they said. "Don't be surprised if she comes a little early." This being my first pregnancy, I had no idea what to expect for the birth. I read every natural birthing book I could get my hands on and decided I wanted to birth at home, in a birth pool. I loved Ina May's quote from her popular *Guide to Childbirth*—"In the medical community birth is something that happens to women . . . In the midwifery community, birth is something women DO." I was set on being in control for this birth and the more I read, the more I felt comfortable about doing it at home. I didn't want drugs imposed on me or to be in a sterile environment surrounded by strangers. I envisioned myself at home, burning incense, candles lit, singing mantras, surrounded by our dogs. Having already been told to prepare for labor in week thirty-six, as the days continued I started becoming more and more anxious to see the baby. I was huge, and now had pelvic pain so intense it was getting difficult to walk. By the time my due date finally rolled around at the end of February, I was so uncomfortable. I couldn't sleep at night, had intense heartburn, and the pelvic and pubic bone pain I'd been experiencing over the last month had intensified to the point that I wasn't even able to get off the couch.

The last days of my pregnancy were some of the most challenging days of my life. I had never been so uncomfortable. Dennis and I did every trick in the book: we went for long walks, I ate spicy food, drank castor oil, ate tons of pineapple, had sex . . . nothing worked. In the back of my mind I knew March 10 was coming, but the idea of another ten days of heavy pregnancy felt unimaginable. The days dragged on, and the midwives started getting worried about my being overdue. "We'll give you a week," they said. "You can go until March seventh, but after that we'll have to induce you and you'll need to have a hospital birth." "But I told you March tenth all along!" I cried. "I'm not having this baby at the hospital. I'm having her at home." There were three midwives working at the center and only one of them agreed to go on with a home birth if I went as far as two weeks overdue. "It better be March tenth," she said. "It will be," I said.

Finally, the day arrived. I woke up giddy with anticipation, like a child on Christmas Day. "Today is the day!" I told Dennis. He yawned, still sleepy, and looked at me. "Okay— just lie back and push then!" he joked. This whole time he'd been pretty ambivalent about my being set on this specific date. "You think you can tell this baby when it's time for her to come out but you can't!" he said, suddenly serious. "It might be today. It might not. You're going to have to let go of control." I knew he was right, but it wasn't easy. I spent the day talking to the baby, immersed in meditation, on my yoga mat, and walking around the house getting everything ready. I was on pins and needles, feeling for any sort of movement or something that might resemble a contraction. Nothing. When afternoon rolled around I started getting anxious—this was supposed to be the day!—and went out to sit on the porch. "Listen, darling. I'm ready for you. Please come out now. You are so loved. We are so ready for you. Today is a perfect day to make your way earth-side!" I felt the baby move, and suddenly heard her talking back. "*No*," she said. I was stunned. I closed my eyes, and when I envisioned the baby I could actually see her with her arms crossed, legs pressing up on the sides of my uterus, face serious. She was pouting! "No," she said again. No? Just no? I couldn't believe it.

The doorbell rang—it was my acupuncturist, Romina. I'd been seeing her consistently every week throughout the pregnancy and had asked her to come over to help get labor started.

She is known on the island as someone who talks to babies—many women see her around the end of their pregnancies to help get labor going. Being with her is like being in the presence of a wise elder, and she'd been a pillar of support for me all throughout the pregnancy. We went upstairs and she started working on me. "Ten days overdue, eh?" she said. "You must be feeling very uncomfortable." I smiled, knowing she knew what I felt. I lay on my side as she put needles in different parts of my body, connecting to energy points known to induce labor. "You're tense today," she said. "Is everything okay?" "It's just important that she comes today," I said. "Why?" Romina asked. "It just is." I told her about wanting to have the home birth and feeling pressured to have labor start so I wouldn't have to go to the hospital, but even as I told the story I knew it was only a small part of the truth. This wasn't about the hospital, or the midwives, or about home birth . . . this was about Andrea. I needed the baby to be born today so I could feel more connected to her. Almost the whole day had passed and I hadn't even spoken to her—actually, I hadn't even thought about her at all. Normally on the anniversary of her death I'd sit down by her altar, or write to her, or try to talk to her, but I was so set on having the birth happen on this day that I'd completely ignored the big, intense wave of grief I could feel now, stuck in the back of my throat. I said nothing and just pushed it away. I didn't want to cry, not now. I had to focus on the baby. Romina continued working on me and went from needles to cupping. As she pulled vacuum-sealed glass vials over my back, I felt a sadness so heavy wash over me that I almost couldn't contain it. I didn't want to feel it. I needed this to be a day of joy, not pain! I wanted so badly to turn everything around, to change the story, to flip the script . . . but as I was lying there, hugging my enormous belly, needles in my feet, I was beginning to realize that maybe, just maybe, that wasn't how life worked. Suddenly, Romina stopped. Very quietly, she put her hands on the sides of my belly and squatted down next to me. An electric wave of energy entered the room and I could feel the hairs on the backs of my arms stand up. For a long time neither of us spoke. Then she stood up and broke the silence. "What happened on this day?" she said. "What do you mean?" I asked. "Something happened on this day. Something painful." I don't know how she knew, but I couldn't hold back the tears anymore. "My best friend died. Three years ago." "On this day?" Romina asked. I nodded. "Yes." "Okay," she said. "Listen. The baby, she sits right beneath your heart. Right here. She feels everything you feel. That pain, in your heart, welling up in the back of your throat? You have to let it out." I was bawling now. The sadness that came pouring out of me was so heavy I just couldn't keep it in. Romina sat down on the bed next to me and held my hand. "This is a day for mourning. It will always be a day of mourning. Birth will come another day. The baby is saying, don't mix the two. She wants her own day, one just for her! Take today to mourn. This baby is not coming out today—I hear her saying 'No.'" She closed her eyes and smiled. "It's funny, I can even see her in there, arms crossed over her chest!" The pain was unbearable. "Keep going," Romina said. "Talk to her. Talk to them both. Let it go. Go into the pain so you can let it go."

I was shaking uncontrollably now, crying intensely. All the

grief and pain I'd held inside, the determination to push away the pain and replace it with something else, came washing over me. Romina lay down on the bed and held me and for the longest time, I just cried.

I stayed there for a long time, holding my hands on my gigantic belly, crying and missing my best friend, longing for my baby girl. At some point I must have fallen asleep because when I woke up, it was dark. I'd slept the whole afternoon. Romina had left—she must have taken the needles out in my sleep. I felt tired but clearheaded. All the anxiousness I'd felt around the birth had washed away. I went out on the balcony. The moon was rising over the desert. She was almost full. I tilted my head back and spoke to Andrea. "I miss you," I said. "I miss you so much. I'm sorry I tried to make your day into something else. It just . . . hurts. You would have been her favorite aunt. It's hard to miss you this much. But I can do it. I can live with missing you. I know that because . . . I am. I miss you every day. And I will for as long as I live."

I realized we can't replace death with birth. They are intertwined, but not interchangeable. Before we can open a new chapter in our lives, we have to take care of the old. The chapters written before come along with us—we can't just let them scatter in the wind. The love we've held and the pain we've felt shape us and become an integral part of who we are. I'd spent months intent on replacing a painful memory with a joyful one, only to realize that if I did, it would have been another loss. No matter how painful, there is also beauty to be found in grief, in feeling everything so intensely that we can't help but share our aching hearts with the world. Grief shows us who we really are.

Andrea's death day will always be a day for mourning and in that moment I knew: I can choose to sit with pain. It doesn't have to consume me. I don't have to fear it, or escape it, or try to replace it. Sitting there under the stars, for the very first time since becoming pregnant, I could feel the presence of both Andrea and the baby. If I just leaned back a little bit, I could almost feel her right there, holding me. "Don't worry, Macha," she whispered. "I'm right here."

I took a deep breath, and as I exhaled, the baby moved. A big, slow, sweeping movement—under my hands, I could feel her turning. Through my tears I broke out in a smile because, again, I could see her. She didn't have her arms crossed over her chest anymore. She was ready.

And so was I.

That night I slept better than I'd had in months, and when I woke up the next day I'd stopped obsessing about the timing of the birth. In a big way, I let go. A day later the moon was full. I woke up at four in the morning with what I intuitively knew were contractions. They were still gentle, caressing me, soft energetic surges running through my body. I kissed Dennis on the cheek and went downstairs, careful not to wake him. I had a feeling he might need his sleep. I lit candles all around the house, burned palo santo, and put on my favorite mantras. I texted my mom, It's starting! It felt so important to share this with her. A part of me wished she was there to hold my hand and guide me through. For hours I danced around the kitchen, twirling my hips, undulating my spine, breathing deeply into the center of my being. The contractions grew more and more intense and when I had to pause to hold on to something to receive the energy, I decided it was time to get Dennis.

I labored for twenty-four hours. It started off gentle but grew more and more intense with each hour's passing. At one point, when I was sure I couldn't take it anymore, Dennis brought me out into the garden. The pain was unbearable and I could feel myself losing my ground. How much longer would this last? Would I actually be able to do this? Dennis held me close. For the longest time we were slow dancing through contractions under the full moon. There was something about being outside . . . The moonlight calmed me. I'd been trying to escape the pain, dreading each contraction as it approached. Standing under the light of the full moon, I could hear Andrea speak to me. "Dive," she said. "Meet it. Feel it. Everything you've ever been through has prepared you for this moment." I was jolted out of the daze I was in and suddenly felt myself transported back to my ayahuasca experience. *The pain is in the resistance. Allowing brings peace. Let. Go.* When the next contraction came, instead of trying to make my way around the pain, I started moving into it. I took a huge breath and stepped toward the fire. Whenever a surge came, instead of escaping it, I went deep inside. Dennis was completely holding me and I could let go in his arms. Strangely, moving toward the pain brought about a way for me to cope, and I felt almost like a surfer, riding a wave. The waves of contractions reminded me of the waves of grief I'd experienced throughout the years and especially the year after Andrea died. I remember walking down the street, feeling completely normal, when suddenly something would remind me of her and grief would hit me so hard that I'd double over and cry in the middle of the sidewalk. Contractions were similar; they'd arrive and hit me hard. There was nowhere to go but within. During one specifically intense surge I realized: this was the gift Andrea truly gave me. The lesson I learned through her, the lesson I've kept learning, was exactly this, to not escape. To sit with pain. To move with it instead of against. This was the lesson that finally settled in me two days earlier, sitting on the balcony. The only way out is through. Standing there in the moonlight, I felt her presence so strongly.

The midwife had been coming over to check in every few hours and had told me at the first checkup that I was four centimeters dilated (which felt like good news!). Now, eighteen hours later, I was sure I was at least eight or nine centimeters along. She had to be coming soon—the pain was otherworldly. The midwife looked at me. "I know this will be disappointing to hear, but you haven't progressed. We're still at four," she said. Something inside of me cracked. I just knew then and there: I needed help. The seventh key of the Path of Love process came to mind: ask for divine help. That was it—I needed help. This was not going to happen at home. I just knew. It was instinctual. I said, "I think we need to go to the hospital. It's not going to happen at home. I want to go. Now." Off to the hospital we went. We got in the car. I was scared that the contractions were going to get much harder as we drove down the bumpy roads from our house, but the strangest thing happened. The moment I got in the car, the moment we left the house and headed for the hospital, something in me completely let go and I was able to actually fall asleep. I'd done something I never do, something I'd struggled with my whole life: I'd asked for help. Going to the hospital, something so common that most women opt for when it comes to giving birth, had been the last thing I wanted and now became a deeply spiritual act. It was an act of giving up, of letting go of control. It was my surrender—cockroaches turning to white doves—it was a giving in to something greater than me. It was prayer. I understood—I couldn't do this on my own. It didn't mean that I couldn't do it without a doctor present, but that I had to surrender to God. I had to let go. I didn't have all the answers. There are certain things books can't teach you. For me, the drive to the hospital was one of the most sacred experiences of my life. I felt like I was buzzing, sparkling with energy and light.

We got to the hospital and it was absolutely quiet. There was not a single other birth happening in the entire place. As soon as we got out of the car contractions started again but the energy completely changed. From intense, loud, overwhelming . . . Everything got so, so quiet. My pain didn't diminish—it was still getting more and more intense—but I could tell things were actually progressing now. I could feel how my body was opening up. Giving up and giving in allowed my body to open. I spent four hours sitting upright in the hospital bed in what felt like a deep, deep meditation. I had more space between contractions, and I was able to remain completely focused and in the moment. Dennis was half asleep on a chair. The room was so silent I could hear my heart beating. Suddenly, I felt like it was time. Changing positions on the bed, I started pushing. It was hard. In many ways, it was harder than the contractions. After what felt like an eternity the midwife exclaimed, "Here she comes! Give me your hands!" And I thought, *My hands?! What?* She guided my hands down. She was coming. Finally, she was coming. With one final push I pulled her out and brought her to my chest. She came out with her eyes wide open. She didn't scream or cry; she just announced her arrival. Her heart beat against mine. She looked at me. All of time stopped.

We locked eyes and I remember thinking: *Oh—There you are. I know you.* I knew right away, this wasn't the first time we'd met. We'd been here many times before.

We named her Lea Luna. Lea for me. Luna for the moon that brought her here and also for Andrea; for the light that follows us even in the dark.

Looking down at her, I knew: it was true, what the shaman had told me. Birthing her was a new beginning and, at the same time, a shedding of all that was old. Her very existence was healing generations of pain I'd been carrying throughout my life. The life purpose I had thought was heavy now felt like the most natural thing in the world. I would do it all again. For her, I'd do it all. My whole life, I'd been so worried about having a baby, about passing on a pain carried through generations. Looking at Lea Luna, I realized I could rest, knowing she would never carry pain that wasn't hers—

how could she? Nothing dark could ever attach to her. She is all light.

In her sleep, she smiled. I held her closer, smelling the top of her head. *Strange*, I thought. *She even smells it. She smells like light.*

She did. Still does. She smells like the full moon.

In the recovery room afterward, I reached for my phone. The last time I was in a hospital bed the number I dialed was Andrea's. She never answered. Now, in a different hospital and another life entirely, my mother picks up right away. She is crying. "Is everything okay? Is she here? Are you alright?" "We're great," I say. I look down at my daughter, laying peacefully in my arms. "Lea, meet Mormor." Through my tears, I can't stop smiling.

We go home and it's not until later, when everything is quiet and we're in bed and Dennis is sleeping and I'm holding our little girl in my arms that I'm able to take it all in. We made it. We made it here. I look down at our perfect daughter. She has fallen asleep with her chubby little cheek pressed against my arm, right on my tattoo that says "I believe in the good things coming." Andrea and I had that song, "Black as Night," on repeat and danced to it more times than I could count during our last days together. She chose the color of her bridesmaid's dress with the song playing in the background. Throughout the last years I've played it obsessively, wanting so badly for the words to become true. I wanted to believe in "the good things coming, coming, coming"—for there to be a life after her death. I wanted to believe things were going to be okay. When I walked down the aisle, the tattoo had just begun to heal and tiny flakes of black ink and skin were falling off my arm, scattering in the wind.

Now here we are, three years later, Lea Luna resting her head on the very same spot. I look down and, just then, in this moment, it dawns on me:

The good things came.

EPILOGUE

March 10, 2019

I'm sitting on the edge of your grave, my bare feet dangling in the empty space that's now filled with dirt and flowers and also your ashes, and the thought of that being true is more than my heart can grasp. You're dead. It's been years but I still don't understand it. Your sister is sprinkling glitter over your urn—a small wooden box that's filled with what was once your body—which we've placed on a little platform six feet below. The glitter is golden and it's spreading everywhere, twirling over my feet, making everything glow with light. Today is the five-year anniversary of your death. Five whole years have passed since the day you left and took so much with you. I missed your first funeral because I was in the hospital recovering from the surgery I had to have because someone decided that your dying meant something had to get cut out of me, too. Doctors I didn't know tried to cut the part of you that's entangled with my being out of my stomach, but they didn't succeed. I have the scars, and even looking at them now, I'm not sure what you were trying to tell me then other than that you were dying and it hurt and you needed me to feel it with you. I thought the pain would kill me but it didn't. It killed you. And now here we are.

It's been five years and your ashes have been on your mother's bedside table this whole time. She can't let you go. None of us can. I don't think we're supposed to. I close my eyes and I can see you dancing. You are always dancing. It's so vivid, so real; if I reach my hands out in front of me I can almost touch you. I open my eyes. Your sister is here. Your mom. Your aunt. Your cousins. Your closest friends. There is so much left here. We are all left, here. I wonder if you see us.

There is a tree above your grave. It's the same kind of tree that suddenly came to life after we buried Pepper; a cherry tree. Except this one is alive already; it's been waiting for you all this time. I drop a yellow rose into your grave and it lands right next to your urn but it remains standing, leaning against you. I look down at my feet. My toes are painted yellow, your favorite color. I feel a wave coming—a big one. It's been five years and still grief takes me by surprise. I'm about to let it take me when, suddenly, everything lights up. The grave, the flowers, my feet, your ashes. The sun has come out from behind the clouds and now everything is shining. I watch the glitter scatter over the earth and remember all the times since you passed that I've felt you here with me. You are the light that bounces off my wedding ring in the midst of a panic attack on a plane. You are my husband's arms, picking me up off the floor. You are the space between my grandmother's breaths. You are my dog who died, and it was nobody's fault. You are my friends, holding me, waiting for the waves to pass. You are my mom, loving me infinitely. You are my daughter, pointing at the moon, smiling at the sky like she has a secret.

You are the light that glitters across the ocean as the sun sets.

Thank you. For everything. For the time we had together. It was short, but it was just enough.

AFTERWORD

I'm sitting at my desk, looking at the cacti sway in the distance through my window. I have a cup of tea by my side, and as usual, Ringo is sleeping by my feet. Dennis is at the studio and Lea is at school (school!); she is four now and goes to a little Montessori a few minutes away. I just watered the vegetable garden, one of the many projects that sprouted in my life in the year and a half since *To Love and Let Go* was released. Where there was once nothing; just a patch of dirt on a neglected side of our house, now grows an abundance of tomatoes, eggplant, kale, and cucumber. Watering the garden every day as I rise has become part of my morning routine. It's 2021 and even though the view of the cacti I see through my window is the same as it always was, it feels like almost everything else has changed.

Writing *To Love and Let Go* was one of the most challenging and healing things I've ever done. It took me years to write the book, and I submitted the final version of the manuscript in spring of 2019. Lea Luna had just turned two at the time and motherhood was just as wonderful as it was all-consuming.

Even though I'd slowed down a ton; spending as much time as I could at home and trading traveling and tours for teaching at our own studio, my life was still moving at an intense pace. Leading back-to-back retreats and teacher trainings for months straight was a regular occurrence, and even though I talked about it a lot I still didn't quite know what "slowing down" truly meant. Looking back at it now; it actually wasn't so much about the things I did or what was on my plate but more about my motivation for *why* I was living my life the way I was. I didn't know it then, but like for so many people across the world, 2020 was about to arrive and teach me a thing or two about life.

At the end of 2019, I was tired. I'd toured the US with this book, teaching yoga in big event halls and hugging as many people as I could in bookstores all across the country. The year had been a flurry of new projects, deadlines, and commitments. Dealing with a cold I just couldn't seem to kick for months, and worse, sensing a loss of inspiration within me, I decided to do something drastic: take a year off. As you know from reading this book, I work a lot. All the time. The idea of taking an entire year to do something else; to explore something different, didn't happen casually. The tiredness I felt was deeper than the kind of tired you feel after having an intense year, or from not having had a day off in a while. I felt tired in my bones. In my soul. I yearned for a year when nothing was expected of me. It didn't come easy, but I made the decision: 2020 would be my year off from everything. A year spent at home. A year of space.

Well. It is true what they say: be careful what you wish for.

Without the slightest inkling of what actually lay ahead, I canceled every commitment I had and started envisioning how special 2020 would be. Finally I'd have the space I always longed for! Things seemed to be perfectly aligned; the business was thriving, I had great relationships with everyone in my family, the studio was doing great. This, I decided, was going to be my year.

Then, like a row of dominoes, things started to fall apart. First, for reasons that felt as obvious as they were hard to swallow, I decided to cut my mother out of my life. It was something I just had to do. A lifetime of codependency with my mom was rearing its true impact on me, and taking the plunge to choose myself above all else was terrifying and liberating all at the same time. Two weeks later, the pandemic hit. From our little island, quiet and still COVID-free, we watched the rest of the world shut down, one country after another. When the first cases started trickling in, Lea got sick with a fever that wouldn't go away and we went through one of the scariest moments of our lives; me having to forcefully hold her down to an examination table, kicking and screaming, as a tall man in a hazmat suit swabbed her nose for COVID-19. This was in the very first weeks, when we were all still terrified for our children, for our loved ones, for ourselves. She tested negative the same week we went into lockdown. We had to close the studio and cancel every retreat we had on the books for a year ahead. We lost more than half of our employees. We almost lost the business. But we had each other.

I think of that first month and all the change I went

through in such a short time; letting go of my mom, facing the pandemic, saying goodbye to so many people that had been constants in my life for so long . . . I was so naive. I thought the virus would be gone in a matter of weeks, and that I'd spend maximum of a few months without my mom. "Everything will be back to normal soon," I thought. As I write this, in many ways I'm glad it isn't. "Normal" wasn't great. It has been a year almost to the day since everything happened and even though the virus is still present in my life, my mom is not.

Setting boundaries is a very, very hard thing to do. For me, never having had any, drawing a line in the sand had less to do with the drama that came along with that relationship and more with me finally making myself the most important person in my own life. Setting a boundary isn't just a "no" to the other person—it's a "yes" to yourself. The moment I started saying yes to myself all the relationships I'd struggled with either resolved themselves naturally, or just fell away. My life is so much easier now. And I'm beginning to learn that like most things, setting boundaries is a practice. We don't wake up one morning and suddenly just know how to do it; we learn by doing. For me, I always had that little voice in the back of my head telling me it was my job to fix other people. That every issue in the world was mine to solve, that every person that needed saving was mine to save. I'd been waiting my whole life for other people to change—"Can't they just step up and do more so I don't have to carry everything on my own?" was a common thought I'd sit with. Turns out, it wasn't until I changed how I acted in relationships that the relationships finally changed. Choosing to not step up and be the rescuer of other people meant other people automatically stepped in. And it left me with time and energy to truly take care of myself! Setting boundaries is something that actually is in our control and in a way, the pandemic taught me how to meet my own needs. All the surface stuff fell away and I got to spend an entire year focusing on what truly mattered: my daughter, my husband, and most of all: myself.

When we went into lockdown, the year of peace and quiet I'd longed for took on a new meaning entirely. The first weeks and months terrified me. Cutting my mom out of my life shook my world—I'd done it once before but only for a short time. This felt different; more solid. I knew I needed space to return to myself, and I knew I wouldn't be able to do it together with her. What I didn't expect was what it would trigger inside of me and that I would have a global pandemic to make all those feelings go up by a million. I felt scared. Alone. Like every constant I'd had in my life went out the window. I'd always felt like losing my mom would be the end of the world. She'd always been at the center of it all; more important than me, even. What would my life be without her? Therapy helped me make sense of a lot of it and the pandemic meant even when I wanted to, I couldn't escape what was happening. Everything became too urgent, too in my face. It wasn't just me living my regular old life dealing with a separation from my mother; it was me facing what felt like the actual end of the world. There was no way around it: I had to face it all. So . . . I did.

I committed to therapy and to spending the year making

myself the most important person in my life. That might sound strange—shouldn't that happen naturally?—but for me it meant a complete shift of perspective in every way. I started prioritizing my self-care in a bigger way than I ever knew was possible. I still had my yoga and meditation practice, and I'd always felt I did a good job at taking care of myself. It turns out it doesn't actually matter how much yoga you practice if at the end of the day, you fall to the bottom of the list of all the people and things you take care of. That's what life had been like for me for so long: I didn't prioritize myself. Everything else felt more important; my family, friends, work, our animals, even the house. "When everything is clean, I'll relax," I'd think. "When all my work is done I'll have more time to focus on myself." Well—that time just never came. I'd squeeze in a yoga practice or a bath at the end of the day but internally, I was still running a hundred miles per hour. The pandemic stopped all of that. Suddenly, there wasn't that much work to do. No parents to worry about. No employees to manage. No big projects to complete. It was just me, Dennis, and Lea and how we filled our days was completely up to us.

In the beginning, every time I'd arrive at a moment of true space it came as a bit of a shock. I was so used to going from thing to thing; task to task; that when suddenly there was nothing left to "do" I'd panic. If the house is clean, and Lea is playing with Dennis outside, and everything is in order and dinner is ready and I have no work to do . . . What next? That question became a big spiritual practice for me. I'd find myself with unexpected windows of space and my mind would immediately go; "What next?" I could go in search of the next thing to "do," but with time I realized that those moments were the gold I'd been searching for my whole life. Every time my mind brought me that question; "What next"—I'd take a deep breath and instead ask myself: "What now?" What if instead of jumping into the next thing, I could practice putting all of my years of yoga into action and arrive here, now? What if I didn't have to jump into the next thing? What if that moment of space was the calm I'd been looking for my entire life? I suddenly had moments trickling in through my day where I would close my eyes, place my hands to my heart, and drop deeply into my body. Nothing to do, nowhere to go. Here, now. The more I practiced present moment awareness in those sudden openings in my day, the more my heart softened. Truth is; there doesn't have to be a "next" task. My life wasn't an out of control freight train I had no ability to stop. I'd been in charge of creating the busyness of my life—and I also had the ability to stop it. Those moments of space were my first, real moments of slowing down. Actually allowing for that space and receiving the calm they brought took real practice. I couldn't just hit the SLOW DOWN button; I had to practice catching those moments and settling into them. I had to allow myself to receive. Little by little, a new level of self-care practice came my way. I committed to fifty consecutive days of Dynamic Meditation. I continued going to therapy, even in weeks when I felt I didn't "need it." I started rising at five a.m. and spent two hours every morning practicing yoga, dancing, and journaling. I picked up a running practice. Where before, I'd always felt there wasn't enough time in the day for me, now I had an abundance of time dedicated to myself. And the best part was: I didn't feel guilty for any of it. Taking care of myself meant I could be a better mom, a better wife, a better friend. Putting myself first changed everything for the better.

After a little while, the rhythm of my life changed entirely. My year of space actually happened. I found myself painting more, reading more, smiling more. Little projects sprouted around the house; some out of joy, some out of fear; because that's the thing about 2020: we enjoyed the little things but we feared the big ones. In all of my slowing down there was still the constant stress of the pandemic looming. One of the greatest joys of my life now, a year later, bloomed not out of love but out of pure panic.

Aruba is such a small island, and it's not self-sustaining. We rely on other countries shipping goods here for survival, and for a while at the very beginning it seemed as if the world was really about to end. Remember all those empty supermarket shelves? The toilet paper shortages? Well, here, when the supermarket shelves ran empty we knew there wasn't a distribution center, or a factory, or a farm, that would eventually provide us with more. There is no farming in Aruba; the island doesn't grow any of its own food. There was a real fear, not just of the pandemic and what it would bring, but of need. The empty shelves at the supermarket triggered a massive fear inside of me. For a long time, I was more terrified of running out of food than I was getting sick. We'd started a small vegetable garden a few months earlier, and although it was something that interested me, I hadn't immersed myself in gardening. I didn't have the time! But now, not knowing if the apocalypse was coming or if we'd have enough food to eat, the garden became the center of my life. In more ways than one, it saved me. Little by little, the garden became the center of my day. I learned about transplanting seedlings and trimming tomato stalks and composting food scraps from the kitchen. I learned that even though the world felt like it was crumbling all around me, there are constants in nature. I could plant a seed and watch it grow. Water my plants and watch them thrive. Harvest my vegetables and turn them into dinner. The garden helped me make sense of things—it became a steady ground in an otherwise unsteady world.

Most of the changes that transpired in my life since *To Love and Let Go* came out happened through that strange mix of love and fear, joy, and panic, and even though there were many moments I'd never choose for myself I am grateful they brought me to where I am now. I trust that there will be a time when this pandemic is behind us, and when that day comes, I hope I'm still gardening. I hope I continue asking myself "What now?" instead of "What next?" I hope I'm still putting myself first.

The other day, cleaning my altar, I paused to read the card Andrea wrote me right before she died. The seven-year anniversary of her passing was just a few days ago and as for every anniversary, she makes her presence known in the most unexpected way. In a strange way, I feel her presence with me now in a stronger way than the years right after she died. Maybe it's the changes I've made in my life; that I finally have the space to listen again. Maybe she was always here exactly the way she is now, I just didn't have the time to talk to her. In the card she wrote me she said "Always remember Your light, your feet in the sand, your EARTH. Take care of that beautiful soul & body"—and it hit me that I'm probably taking her advice for the first time just now. I stared at those words on that card for years but writing these words, here, now, seven years later, I can feel the truth of her message in my body. I put my hands to the earth every day in the garden. I'm taking care of my body, and my soul. I'm listening.

While looking for a photo of Andrea to post on Instagram I found a video from our time at Envision Festival; one I almost never watch. We're lying in a big net tied between trees, listening to an acoustic set in the village. I'm mostly filming the stage but about thirty seconds in, I turn the camera toward Andrea and for just a moment the video captures her—she smiles at me, clapping her hands and moving her body with the music. It's a beautiful moment and the video captures it so well, but the whole thing is turned sideways. I couldn't figure out how to edit it so I ended up not posting the video but chose a photo from another moment instead.

Later that evening I went out to meditate under the stars— it had been a full day and before bed I found myself feeling sad that I hadn't carved out more space to sit in meditation and talk to her. I walked out onto the patio and sat down under the faint light of the moon. Remembering the video I watched earlier in the day, I pulled my phone out to watch it again. I pressed pause right on the frame that shows her face; smiling, a twinkle in her eyes, and I was hit with the enormity of how much I still miss her. The finality of her death and the fact that no matter what I do, I'll never get a new moment with her again, is still hard for me to accept. *I'll never see a new version of us again*, I thought. I'd give anything for a fresh perspective, a new moment with her. I sat there for a long time, crying my eyes out, looking at that moment of her frozen in time. When I had no more tears to cry I found myself picking up my phone, opening Instagram. There was a new message at the top of my DM's from a person I didn't know. "Hey," the person wrote. "I know you get a lot of messages and you probably won't see this one either, but every year on the anniversary of your friend's death I write you. I have a beautiful photo of the two of you from the festival, maybe this is the year you will see it." I can tell that every year on March 10, there has been a new message sent that I've never seen. I click "open" and suddenly, all of time stops. The screen fills with that exact moment of us—a new perspective of it I've never seen. It's Andrea and me together, side by side, resting in that big hammock, looking out at the scene. The photo is taken from the ground up; a new angle, and it makes it feel like a new moment entirely. Like I was gifted a new memory with her. I look at the time. It's 11:59 p.m.

She always comes to me when I need her. She's always right on time.

ACKNOWLEDGMENTS

I wrote the first words of what would become the book you are now holding in your hands sitting on a dock looking out at the ocean, my stomach wrapped in bandages. It was my husband, Dennis, who told me earlier that day: don't dwell in the dark. Go sit in the light and talk to her. So I did. I sat down in the light of the setting sun, notebook in my lap, and I started writing. Every word I've written since then has come as a result of his unwavering support. It would take me five years to finish this book and I never in a million years would have been able to do it without him. Dushi—I love you so much. Thank you for everything.

To the many, many people, who have supported me from afar and who continue to cheer me on. To my students, who are also my greatest teachers. To every single person who listens to the podcast, follows my journey online, and who reads my words every day: thank you. From the bottom of my heart, I am forever grateful for this community and for the magic it continues to create at every turn.

To my editor, Lauren Spiegel, who believed in this book

even when I didn't. Thank you for the countless hours spent pouring over these pages and for continuing to remind me that it was a story that needed to get told.

I owe a big thank you to my dear friend and agent, Rob Koslowsky, who's been there since the very beginning. You've supported me since long before it made any sense—I am so thankful for your presence in my life. It's almost time to retire! The Caribbean awaits.

To Angela Rydén, our saving grace, for steering the ship that is Yoga Girl® as I spent months putting everything else aside to finish this book. Without you, I wouldn't be here, writing these words. I am forever grateful for your heart, your dedication, and your hard work. Thank you for giving me the gift of structure and peace of mind so that I can continue doing what I do, every day.

To Olivia and Daniella, for holding my hand and for guiding me throughout it all. Without you, I would never have been able to put the pieces of my broken heart back together. Thank you for showing me the meaning of sisterhood, every day. You are the stars that light up my universe. I love you more than I could ever put into words.

I want to thank the friends who were there in the hard moments, the beautiful moments, and the wonderfully mundane ones in between. To Rose, for reminding me to breathe and helping me see the light. To Jessica, who brings sunshine wherever she goes. To Mathias, who is far away but always close. To Laura, who might be little, but has the biggest heart I've ever known. To Jen, who always tells it like it is. To Mikaela, for helping me notice the signs. And to Pati, who always gets it. I love you so.

To Jess and Courtney, the best assistants I've ever had. My life would be so gray without you! To Margaret Riley King, my literary agent, for connecting the dots and helping me make this book a reality. To Amelie Rehnvall for being a rock and for holding down the fort for so long. Many chapters of this book were written thanks to her. To Robin Gaby Fisher, thank you for your guidance and help in getting this book across the finish line.

To Maja and her little mountain. To Ash and Pumpkin. To Mignon, Ashley, Josh, and Lindsey: I love you.

To Luigi and Josh, Topsy and Bushman, for being the glue that holds our family time together. To Shubhaa, who changed my life, and to Talib, who has taught me so much. To Rafia, for giving me the tools to let go and for helping me write about it.

A Doña Patricia, Juliana, Luisa, Sebastian y Doña Magali— gracias por todo. Son mi segunda familia, mi segundo hogar. Siempre los amare.

The biggest thank you to Ludvig, Katja, Hedda, Emelie, and Maia. You have my whole heart. To Niklas and Mikaela, and the little one on the way. To my grandparents and their parents, too. To my aunts. To Marianne and the many strong women who paved the way long before I was born.

To my mom and dad, who are now Mormor and Morfar; the best parents I could have ever asked for. I love you infinitely. Thank you for giving me the perfect balance of the gifts and challenges I needed to get to where I am today. Thank you for giving me life, for loving me so, and for parenting me the way no one else could have. I wouldn't change a thing.

And finally, to Lea Luna. My little moon. I didn't know it but I waited for you my whole life. Thank you for choosing me to be your mom and for picking the perfect moment to arrive.

ABOUT THE AUTHOR

Swedish native and *New York Times* bestselling author Rachel Brathen is a world-renowned yoga instructor who teaches workshops and leads yoga retreats around the globe. Find her on Instagram: @yoga_girl and at www.yogagirl.com.

ALSO BY
RACHEL BRATHEN

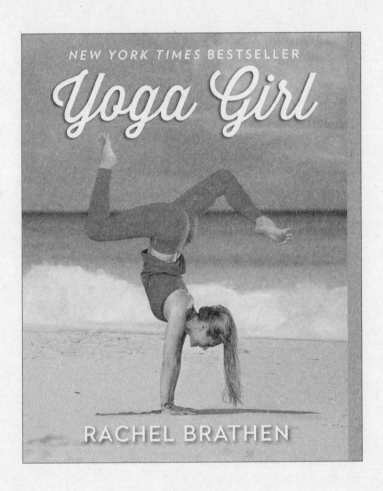

69710